Harnessing Digital Technology and Data for Nursing Practice

Harnessing Digital Technology and Data for Nursing Practice

Edited by

NATASHA PHILLIPS, PhD, RN, DipHe, Bsc(Hons)
Honorary Professor of Nursing and Digital Health
University of Salford, Manchester
United Kingdom
Founder Future Nurse, London
United Kingdom

GEMMA STACEY, PhD, MN, RN, PGCHE, PFHEA
Deputy Chief Executive Officer
Florence Nightingale Foundation, London
United Kingdom

DAWN DOWDING, PhD, RN, FAAN, FIAHSI
Professor in Clinical Decision Making
Division of Nursing, Midwifery and Social Work
The University of Manchester, Manchester
United Kingdom

ELSEVIER

Notices

Practitioners and researchers must always rely on their own experience and knowledge in evaluating and using any information, methods, compounds or experiments described herein. Because of rapid advances in the medical sciences, in particular, independent verification of diagnoses and drug dosages should be made. To the fullest extent of the law, no responsibility is assumed by Elsevier, authors, editors or contributors for any injury and/or damage to persons or property as a matter of products liability, negligence or otherwise, or from any use or operation of any methods, products, instructions, or ideas contained in the material herein.

ISBN: 978-0-443-11160-0

Content Strategist: Robert Edwards
Content Project Manager: Abdus Salam Mazumder
Design: Ryan Cook
Marketing Manager: Deborah Watkins

Printed in India at Replika Press Pvt Ltd.

Last digit is the print number: 9 8 7 6 5 4 3 2 1

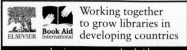

Working together
to grow libraries in
developing countries

www.elsevier.com • www.bookaid.org

CONTENTS

When I started working in healthcare technology as a nurse informaticist almost 40 years ago (yes, in 1984!), the concept was new and not many healthcare professionals participated. It was much more common for analysts and developers to have a computer technology background and no clinical knowledge. It would take almost a decade for the integration of these two disciplines to become commonplace and for all to realize that technology is but the means to an end and not a 'magic pill' to transform the healthcare system. Emphasis changed from technology itself to a focus on understanding the clinical practice changes, defining expected patient outcomes, applying user-centred design, outlining streamlined clinician workflows and planning effective and efficient system implementations. Today, digital technologies and data science are considered foundational tools to transform the healthcare system. There are thousands of doctors and nurses working in technology roles around the world, ensuring the focus is on the care process and not on the technology.

The importance of nursing involvement in technology implementation and adoption cannot be overstated. Nurses know what it is like to be on the frontlines of patient care, whether in a doctor's office, hospital, long-term care facility, rehabilitation clinic, or a patient's home. Having the breadth and depth of clinical knowledge and understanding clinical practice workflows, nurses can help others understand the value of technology, and how it will impact patient care. Nurses understand the continuum of care, both by practicing in multiple venues as well as by working with patients at different points in their care journey. This gives them a unique perspective on the use of technology to support good healthcare and ensure a smooth patient experience. They know what it is like not to have care continuity across the continuum or not to have the information needed at each transition of care. Nurses are used to working in teams and thus, have a good understanding of what each person on the healthcare team and across the healthcare continuum is working on, from doctors and pharmacists to dieticians and physical therapists. As such, the nurse understands not only the practice change being facilitated by the technology, but also the impact it will have on each care team member, as well as the role of each member in its successful implementation.

Nurses also promote patients' greater understanding and use of digital technology for their own health and healthcare. As the most trusted profession (U.K. Ipsos Index 2022 and U.S. Gallup Poll 2023), nurses promote patients' use of technology to expand engagement in their own care – a role that involves both opportunity and responsibility. It is important to note that over 99% of patients' lives and activities occur outside of healthcare facilities, when no healthcare professional is present. Therefore, to effectively achieve health outcome improvements, patients and families must become an integral part of the care team, with access to their health information, to participate in their wellness, prevention, early detection, disease management and illness care. Nurses serve as patient advocates, encouraging the adoption of these collaborative practices. Patients and families also need health education services delivered in a patient-appropriate learning environment and format, and nurses have extensive knowledge in patient education methods and tools. The power of the patient in this participatory/partnership role is supported and augmented by technology to create person-centred care and outcome improvement.

The advancement of technology has opened up opportunities to provide care anytime, anywhere – and there is little question that both patients and professionals are increasingly drawn to the concept of virtual healthcare services. This includes 'visits' using communication technologies such as email, phone, and videoconferencing, as well as telehealth technologies for remote monitoring and management of conditions or chronic diseases. This, coupled with patients using portals and mobile apps, creates a new ecosystem for nurses and their patients to interact. Care coordination between venues of care and across the continuum will be directly impacted in a positive way and support health management of the population. As nurses have the primary responsibility of coordinating care and helping patients navigate the complexities of the healthcare system, this will be a way for them to extend their reach to more patients and to improve the quality of the care provided to each patient. Nurses can more easily close care gaps for preventive and disease management services, monitor patients' conditions while they live their lives and not just when they visit a healthcare facility, and provide consulting and educational services.

Data science is one specific technology breakthrough that is making a significant impact on healthcare and helping create a learning health system. It provides a unique ability and opportunity to capture and derive the benefits from data – to translate the seemingly independent pieces of data into meaningful conclusions that, if applied and implemented correctly, can improve the health of individuals and populations, and tailor healthcare to individual patient needs. Again, nurses have an important role to play. Once organizations aggregate relevant health data, nurses can identify practices that measurably impact care and outcomes. Understanding data to identify what does and does not work, or what does and does not produce measurable quality improvement, allows nurses to avoid not only unnecessary interventions, but also practices that might create adverse events. Once collected, the data is mined and researched, correlated and linked to improved outcomes, then iterated back into practice, far faster than ever before possible. It can be built into the patients' electronic health records using order sets, care plans, documentation templates and clinical decision support, making it easy to do the right thing and 'hard-wiring' the new evidence-based best practice. This is one of the most transformative impacts of technology in the healthcare environment over the past decade – the ability to iterate knowledge from quality improvement and research studies back into practice in a timeframe that was unheard of even 10 years ago!

Healthcare is also currently adapting to a wealth of new patient-generated data, which is impacting the data lifecycle as well. Patient-generated data will have a dramatic and ongoing effect on healthcare research, as it captures activities from outside the healthcare facilities where patients live their daily lives. Capturing the social determinants of health and other non-healthcare-facility data is important to understand the overall health outcomes of individuals and populations.

Today, the field of nursing informatics continues to evolve. Given the importance I describe for the involvement of nurses in healthcare technology, what nursing roles and contributions can be expected in the next 20 years to harness digital technology and data science for nursing practice? To answer these questions, the editors invited nursing informatics leaders to share their thoughts on how digital technology and data science will impact person-centred practice, the creation of a digitally ready workforce, digitally enabled nursing/midwifery practice, and digital innovation/research. Nursing professionals are the foundation of care delivery, the integrators of patient care – and in this role, will increasingly require advanced knowledge and expert use of technology. To the authors, editors, and publishers of this book – and to all nursing informatics professionals – thank you for leading the way.

Judy Murphy, DN (hon), RN, FACMI, LFHIMSS, FAAN
Former Chief Nursing Officer, IBM Global Healthcare
Former Chief Nursing Officer, Office of the National Coordinator for Health IT,
at the U.S. Dept of Health & Human Services
Minneapolis, Minnesota, United States

Helen Balsdon, RN, MSc
Interim Chief Nursing Information Officer
Transformation Directorate,
NHS England, London
United Kingdom

Jen Bichel-Findlay, HScD, MN, MPH, GDipN, BAppSc, DipAppSc, RN, FACN, FACHI, AFCHSM
Honorary Associate
Faculty of Health
University of Technology Sydney, Ultimo
New South Wales
Australia
Chair, Nursing and Midwifery Digital Health
  Network
Australasian Institute of Digital Health,
  Melbourne, Victoria
Australia

Antonia Brown, RN, DN, PGDip, QN
Deputy Chief Nursing Information Officer
Digital Transformation
Sussex Community NHS Foundation Trust,
  Brighton
United Kingdom

Holly Carr, BSc Nursing (Child)
Associate Chief Nursing Information Officer
Digital Nursing Team
NHS Transformation Directorate,
  NHS England, Leeds
United Kingdom

Louise Cave, BNurs Adult (Hons)
Florence Nightingale Digital Leadership
  Fellow
Transformation Directorate
NHS England, London
United Kingdom
Cerner Divisional Operations Transformation
  Manager
The Hillingdon Hospital, London
United Kingdom

Aaron Conway, BN Hons, PhD, RN
Conjoint Senior Research Fellow
School of Nursing
Queensland University of Technology and
  The Prince Charles Hospital, Brisbane
Australia

Helen Crowther, RN
National Digital Primary Care Nurse Lead
  NHS England, London
United Kingdom

Jo Dickson, MSc, RN
Chief Nurse
Clinical directorate
NHS Digital, Leeds
United Kingdom

Dawn Dowding, PhD, RN, FAAN, FIAHSI
Professor in Clinical Decision Making
Division of Nursing, Midwifery and Social
  Work
The University of Manchester, Manchester
United Kingdom

Loretto Grogan, RGN, MSc
Chief Nursing and Midwifery Information
  Officer
Health Service Executive, Dublin
Ireland

Sarah Anne Hanbridge, DipN, BA (Hons) PGCE MA
Chief Clinical Information Officer
Digital Services
Leeds Teaching Hospital, Leeds
United Kingdom

Nicholas R. Hardiker, PhD, RN, CMgr, FACMI, FHEA, FAAN
Dean and Professor of Nursing & Health
  Informatics
School of Human & Health Sciences
University of Huddersfield, Huddersfield
United Kingdom

Stacey Hatton, BSc (Hons), MSc
Chief Nursing Information Officer
University Hospitals of Derby and Burton,
    Derby
United Kingdom

Vanessa Heaslip, PhD, MA, BSc(hons), DipHe, RN, DN
Professor of Nursing and Healthcare Equity
School of Health and Society
University of Salford, Salford
United Kingdom
Adjunct Professor of Public Health
Social Work Department
University of Stavanger, Stavanger
Norway

Debbie Holley, PhD, FRSA, PFHEA, NTF
Professor of Learning Innovation
Department of Nursing Sciences
Faculty of Health and Social Sciences
Bournemouth University, Bournemouth
United Kingdom

Betina Idnay, PhD, RN
Postdoctoral Research Fellow
Department of Biomedical Informatics
Columbia University, New York
United States

Gillian Janes, PhD, RGN, MA, BSc (Hons), SFHEA
Associate Clinical Fellow
Nursing
Manchester Metropolitan University,
    Manchester
United Kingdom
Honorary Associate Professor
Centre for Health Systems and Safety Research
Macquarie University, Sydney
Australia

Aaron Jones, RN, DipHe, GradDip Crit Care, MClinEd, FACN
Chief Nursing and Midwifery Information
    Officer
Digital Health and Innovation
Sydney Local Health District, Camperdown
New South Wales
Australia
Adjunct Associate Professor
Faculty of Medicine and Health
University of Sydney, Camperdown
New South Wales
Australia

Henrietta Mbeah-Bankas, MSc, PGCert, BSc (Hons), DipHe, RMN
Head of Blended Learning
Workforce, Training and Education
    Directorate
NHS England
United Kingdom

Tracie Miles, PhD, RGN
Associate Director of Nursing
South West Genomic Medicine Service
    Alliance, NHS
United Kingdom
Honorary Lecturer
University West of England (Genomics in
    Nursing & Midwifery), Bristol
United Kingdom

Sarah Newcombe, RN (child), BSc (Hons), PGDip
Chief Nursing Information Officer
Great Ormond Street Children's Hospital and
    London Region NHS England
United Kingdom

Siobhan O'Connor, BSc, CIMA CBA, BSc, RN, PhD
Senior Lecturer
Division of Nursing, Midwifery and Social
    Work
The University of Manchester, Manchester
United Kingdom

Laura-Maria Peltonen, PhD, RN, FEANS, FIAHSI
Adjunct professor
University Research Fellow
Department of Nursing Science
University of Turku, Turku
Finland

Natasha Phillips, PhD, DipHe, Bsc (Hons)
Honorary Professor of Nursing and Digital
    Health
University of Salford, Manchester,
United Kingdom
Founder Future Nurse, London
United Kingdom

Dione Rogers, RN, BSc, MSc
Chief Nursing Informatics Officer/ Deputy
    Chief Nurse
Barking Havering and Redbridge University
    Hospitals, London
United Kingdom

Charlene Esteban Ronquillo, RN, PhD
Assistant Professor
School of Nursing, Faculty of Health and
    Social Development
University of British Columbia Okanagan,
    Kelowna, BC
Canada

Gemma Stacey, PhD, MN, RN, PGCHE, PFHEA
Deputy Chief Executive Officer
Florence Nightingale Foundation, London
United Kingdom

**Emma Stanmore, PhD, MReS, BNurs (Hons),
DN, RN**
Reader and Healthy Ageing Research Group
    Lead
PGR Tutor
Business Engagement Lead in DNMSW
Director KOKU Health
The University of Manchester, Manchester
United Kingdom

Gillian Strudwick, RN, PhD, FAMIA, FCAN
Senior Scientist and Chief Clinical
    Informatics Officer
Centre for Addiction and Mental Health,
    Toronto
Canada
Associate Professor
Institute of Health Policy, Management and
    Evaluation
University of Toronto, Toronto
Canada

Cristina M. Vasilica, PhD, FHEA
Associate Professor in Digital Health and
    Head of Digital Education
School of Health & Society
University of Salford, Greater Manchester
United Kingdom

Lisa Ward, RGN, MA, BA(Hons)
Associate Director of Nursing (Patient Safety)
    and Chief Nursing Information Officer
County Durham and Darlington NHS
    Foundation Trust
United Kingdom

Emily Wells, RN, PGDip, NMP
Deputy Chief Nursing Information Officer
Digital Health
Norfolk and Norwich University Hospitals
    NHS Foundation Trust
United Kingdom

Jessica Williams, RN, MSc
Principal Genetic Counsellor
Wessex Clinical Genetics Service, Princess
    Anne Hospital, Southampton
United Kingdom

VIDEO TABLE OF CONTENTS

A suite of videos exploring the themes and content within the chapters are available on the Evolve site: http://evolve.elsevier.com/Phillips/digital/

We are facing a global challenge of increased demand for healthcare by an aging population, and we have insufficient workforce to meet these needs. Digital technologies and data science are powerful tools in meeting this challenge, and models of care delivery are changing to incorporate these. As nurses who are contributing to leading the digital transformation of healthcare practice, education and research, we are urging you, the global nursing community, to engage in this agenda. We believe that digitally enabled care has the potential to reconnect nurses with the joy of practice, provided they are equipped with the digital literacy to maximise the benefits and are integral to the development, design and implementation of digital solutions. This book is for all nurses who want to know more about how they can take an active role in ensuring that digital technologies and data science positively impact nursing practice. The case studies shared throughout the book offer examples of what good looks like and provide a blueprint for things to consider and apply to your practice setting. While written by nurses for nurses, the content covered is relevant to and can be applied by midwives and all healthcare professionals.

When digitally enabled person-centred practice is at the heart of nursing and acts as a key driver for new models of care delivery, the shape of the workforce will look different. The nurse of the future will be adept at using health data and advanced clinical insights to make informed decisions. They will communicate with people in a variety of ways, both virtually and in person, and people will have much greater control over, and access to, their own medical records and health data. Technological advances will free up nurse time, for example, by reducing the burden of administrative tasks, increasing the freedom of working locations and ultimately preventing people from becoming ill. However, this will not mean a need for fewer clinicians. This will enable nurses to realise the benefits of the opportunities that new digital approaches provide by engaging with service users holistically and setting aside time for continuous learning.

The contribution of nurses is vital for effective digital transformation. Without it, there is a risk that the accelerated adoption of digital health will have a negative impact on the ability of nurses to deliver care and support health and wellbeing. Nurses suggest that they face the following challenges with digital health:

- Digital technologies are not well designed and cause more work for nurses, thereby affecting their ability to join care across different care settings and to deliver person-centred care that is safe and of high quality.
- Systems are not well connected, and this lack of interoperability affects the ability to share information and creates duplicative work for nurses.
- Low confidence in sharing data and reassuring the public about data security.
- Lack of education at pre- and post-registration to enable nurses to work with technology and handle data to support care.
- Digital technologies often reinforce exclusion of staff, marginalised groups, and communities.

With a surge in remote monitoring and telehealth, the Covid-19 pandemic has demonstrated the ability of nurses to rapidly transform and adopt new ways of working. There is evidence that in some areas, nurses are already taking a leading role in digital healthcare. This book offers the theory, evidence and tools to increase your confidence to lead and to realise how your expertise is integral to ensuring that digital healthcare becomes the enabler to person-centred practice.

PERSON-CENTRED PRACTICE AND DIGITAL TRANSFORMATION

Person-centred practice is an approach established through the formation and fostering of healthful relationships between care providers and people accessing services, including the other people significant to them in their lives. It is under-pinned by values of mutual respect and the individual right to self-determination and understanding and is enabled by cultures of empowerment that foster continu-ous approaches to practice development and quality enhancement (McCormack and McCance 2017). Maximising the benefits of technology, data and information has the potential to enhance the art of person-centred practice and to enable this practice in the context of integrated care. While emerging new technology and digi-tal innovation creates significant opportunities for improvements in person-centred care, these come with a range of challenges and barriers that need to be addressed in order to realise these benefits over the next 20 years.

Many of the key aims of person-centred integrated care can be effectively facili-tated by technology and data. The sharing of population health data and single digital health records, in turn, enabled by robust data governance policies and infrastruc-ture, can support collaborative working across system geographies. Technological opportunities, such as telemedicine, virtual wards and remote monitoring, can enable more personalised care delivered closer to home. Empowering technology, such as self-monitoring wearable devices, patient portals and accessible health pro-motion apps, can increase patient self-management and community engagement. The combined effect of these developments can serve to improve professional qual-ity of life, with nurses able to draw increased satisfaction from more meaningful clinical interactions due to time released from administrative tasks and better infor-mation sharing across sectors.

The roles and functions of the nursing workforce will need to change over the next 20 years in order to realise the benefits of these technological developments for healthcare systems, service users and professionals. This will be underpinned by a philosophical and cultural shift from treating illness to enabling health. The power dynamic between 'professional' and 'patient' will change from paternalism to part-nership, as patients are informed and empowered by the information they can hold about themselves and the democratisation of knowledge. Nurses as care partners will need to develop competence in developing meaningful relationships based on empathy and compassion in the challenging context of virtual interactions, as well as competence in interpreting and using real-time patient analytics to support people in making their own informed decisions about personalised care. The professional's role will be that of a co-navigator of care rather than a prescriber, and this may come with increased risks associated with the potential for patient decisions that are not aligned with the professional's view.

Nurses will also become facilitators of good population health. Increasingly accessible population health data in an integrated care context presents an opportunity for healthcare to re-focus on prevention. Professionals will need to work with people to manage their own health conditions by supporting them to access new technology.

DRIVERS FOR DIGITAL TRANSFORMATION

Globally, it is recognised that digital healthcare is fundamental to healthy populations and there is a desire to address the widespread variation in digital maturity. Thus, the World Health Organization has made digital healthcare a strategic priority for delivery of the Sustainable Development Goals (WHO 2020). Nurses have a vital role in delivering this strategy for digital healthcare.

In England, the emergence of digital healthcare has been slow despite significant investment. While electronic health records (EHRs) have been universally adopted in primary care, enabled by various policy initiatives, much of secondary care remains on paper. The National Programme for Information Technology (NPfIT), established with the aim of delivering a fully digitised National Health Service (NHS) with a national EHR, was shut down 10 years after having failed in this ambition. It has been argued this was due to over-centralisation and an overfocus on the technical aspects of change with a lack of attention to service change and clinical engagement (Greenhalgh et al. 2011). Twenty years on, the digital landscape has shifted significantly and this is captured in numerous policy documents and high-profile reports like the Wachter (2016) and Topol (Health Education England 2019) reviews.

In contrast, the HITECH Act (2009) in the United States led to widespread adoption of EHRs. However, criticisms levied at this approach suggest a limited focus on user-centred design that has increased the workload of all clinicians, including nurses, and in some instances, even created patient safety risks.

DEVELOPMENT OF A SPECIALIST WORKFORCE IN DIGITAL NURSING (NURSING INFORMATICS)

Nurses who use technology or computers to help process and communicate information or data are known as practicing 'nursing informatics' (Saba 2001). Florence Nightingale is widely considered to be the first nursing informatician (Betts and Wright 2020). Through her use of data and illustrations, devising the use of coxcomb to illustrate the causes and rates of death of soldiers during the Crimean War, she pioneered a data-driven approach to improving nursing practice (Betts and Wright 2020).

Whilst computer technology was introduced into healthcare environments as early as the 1950s, it was only in the 1970s that the nursing informatics community began to develop internationally. Early computer applications in nursing included systems for care planning and documentation with the aim of reducing documentation burden whilst improving the quality and completeness of the plan (Ozbolt and Saba 2008). Other early research focused on how to represent nursing knowledge and develop decision support (Ozbolt and Saba 2008). In 1982, the Nursing Informatics working group for the International Medical Informatics Association (IMIA) held its first conference in London, UK and, since then, has served as an international focus for activities in nursing informatics (Saba 2001). Nursing informatics was formally defined in 1989 as 'a scientific discipline uniting nursing science, information science, and computer science to manage and process nursing data, information, and knowledge in support of nursing practice' (Graves and Corcoran 1989). Nursing informatics was identified as a nursing specialty by the American Nurses Association (ANA) in 1992 and a third edition of the Scope and Standards of Practice related to the specialty was published in 2022 (American Nurses Association 2022).

Since the early days, the work of nurses in the field of informatics has furthered our knowledge and understanding of how to develop systems to enable the capture of data to inform nursing practice, and how to use that data to support practice. For example, developing common classifications or nursing-specific languages that ensure nursing practice is identified and codified in electronic systems (Saba 2001). Nurses have also been involved in the development and evaluation of applications used to support nursing care and practice. In the United States, the specialty of nursing informatics is well developed, with a number of educational courses designed to enable nurses to meet the scope and standards of practice outlined by the ANA, and with nurses working in education, research and practice in the field of digital and nursing. Understanding the underpinning knowledge and research conducted by the early nursing informaticists, and how this underpins the development of nursing and digital transformation going forward, is crucial to ensure that nurses are positively impacted by and contribute to the digital transformation of healthcare.

OVERVIEW OF THE BOOK

This book will enable nurses to maximise the opportunities that digital transformation presents for the progression of nursing practice and, ultimately, for better patient outcomes. It will also support readers to navigate the challenges associated with engaging with large-scale, system-wide change that will impact every nurse across all sectors, settings and specialities.

Section 1 focuses on person-centred practice and situates the learning in the history, underpinning theory and current trends of nursing care to demonstrate the way in which digital transformation and technological advances remain integral to progressing the art of practice. We critically explore the changing nature of the relationship between people accessing and delivering care, as people have increasing access and control over their health data. We expand on this to address the potential exclusion and exacerbation of health inequalities that could occur through digitally enabled practices. We also consider the opportunities of reaching to previously dis-advantaged groups by utilising innovative digital engagement strategies and big data to target our population health initiatives. This will only be possible with a com-mitment to meaningful input from people and professionals who are the users of the technology and data from the outset of the design process. The principles and values of user-centred design are therefore essential to ensuring a digitally enabled person-centred practice.

Section 2 focuses on the development of the nursing workforce to practice in, and lead, the development of digital healthcare. The increasing use of digital technolo-gies and data science in healthcare has led to the need for nurses to develop new knowledge and skills to deliver safe, effective, person-centred practice. However, evidence shows that nursing practice is often hindered by poor technology that increases their workload. Arguably, nurses need to take up leadership roles in digital healthcare across both policy and practice and from inception to implementation of digital solutions to address this challenge. This section examines the breadth of lead-ership required from specialist digital nursing roles to the wider collective leadership required to achieve large-scale transformation across complex systems. Digital tech-nologies advance at rapid pace and a culture of innovation is required where nurses can identify practice issues and innovate to resolve these. There is an opportunity for nurses to act as entrepreneurs, develop these ideas and take them to market for the benefit of patients and staff. This will only be possible in organisations and systems that support nurses to develop entrepreneurial skills.

Section 3 focuses on how nursing practice is rapidly evolving to encompass the use of a breadth of technologies and data to inform care delivery, operational man-agement and population health. At the most fundamental level, this entails docu-menting nursing care in EHRs; however, it increasingly involves new technologies and ways of working. The pandemic has led to a rapid rise in remote care enabled by wearables and virtual consultations. As digital healthcare evolves, clinical decision support underpinned by algorithms will increasingly become integral to practice. The nurse will have a key role in managing risk and ensuring that digital makes care safer. In addition, as nurses increasingly work in a large digital ecosystem where the pace and volume of data sharing rapidly grows, issues of information governance and cybersecurity will be more prevalent and complex. This section examines all these areas and their implications for nurses and nursing practice.

Section 4 discusses how using digital technologies can enable the transforma-tion of nursing practice. With the advent of digital systems, nurses have access to vast quantities of data about the care they provide and the outcomes for patients. Improvement science methodologies are an established approach to managing change and improving care. We discuss how these approaches are used to enable effective digital transformation, ensuring that the process is managed as a qual-ity improvement or change project, rather than a purely technical implementa-tion. Data is used across health and care organisations in a variety of ways, such as to inform quality and safety monitoring, performance and compliance, quality improvement, organisational change and, increasingly, management of population health. We explore the uses of data for nursing practice and the implications of the data for future practice. Finally, we explore the role of research and digital nursing practice. Digital systems support nurse researchers, as well as provide data to answer clinical practice questions developed by researchers. Understanding if and how the innovations developed as part of digital nursing practice impact nurses and those they care for is a growing area of research, which will ensure that future practice is evidence based.

In section 5, readers will embark on a journey of discovery into the future of nursing, where digital technologies and data-driven insights are revolutionising healthcare delivery. By comprehending the nuances of genomics, remote care, virtual wards, AI, and other digital tools, nurses can equip themselves to thrive in this dynamic and transformative healthcare landscape. The knowledge gained from this section will empower nurses to be leaders in the digital age, championing person-centered care through innovation and technology.

As nurses practicing across the world, the digital transformation agenda is relevant to every one of us. We have an important role to play in leading and shaping the way forward. We cannot be passive recipients of technology. As we embark on this pivotal time for our profession, we invite you to consider your role in maximising the benefits of digitally enabled practice for the people and communities you support, your teams and your students.

References

American Nurses Association, 2022. Nursing informatics: scope and standards of practice, third ed. American Nurses Association, Silver Spring.

Betts, H.J., Wright, G., 2020. 200 Years since the birth of nursing informatics? In: The importance of health informatics in public health during a pandemic, vol. 272. IOS Press, pp. 28–32. https://doi.org/10.1016/j.ijnurstu.2021.104153.

Graves, J.R., Corcoran, S., 1989. The study of nursing informatics. Image J Nurs. Sch. 21 (4), 227–231. https://doi.org/10.1111/j.1547-5069.1989.tb00148.x.

Greenhalgh, T., Russell, J., Ashcroft, R.E., et al., 2011. Why national eHealth programs need dead philosophers: Wittgensteinian reflections on policymakers' reluctance to learn from history. Milbank Q. 89 (4), 533–563.

Health Education England, 2019. The Topol review: Preparing the healthcare workforce to deliver the digital future. Available at: https://topol.hee.nhs.uk/wp-content/uploads/HEE-Topol-Review-2019.pdf.

McCormack, B., McCance, T., 2017. Person-centred practice in nursing and health care: theory and practice. Wiley-Blackwell, Oxford.

Ozbolt, J.G., Saba, V.K., 2008. A brief history of nursing informatics in the United States of America. Nur. Outlook. 56 (5), 199–205.e2. https://doi.org/10.1016/j.outlook.2008.06.008.

Saba, V.K., 2001. Nursing informatics: yesterday, today and tomorrow. Int. Nurs. Rev. 48 (3), 177–187. https://doi.org/10.1046/j.1466-7657.2001.00064.x.

Wachter, R.M., 2016. Making IT work: harnessing the power of health information technology to improve care in England. Available at: https://assets.publishing.service.gov.uk/government/uploads/system/uploads/attachment_data/file/550866/Wachter_Review_Accessible.pdf.

World Health Organization, 2020. Global strategy on digital health 2020–2025. Available at: https://www.who.int/docs/default-source/documents/gs4dhdaa2a9f352b0445bafbc79ca799dce4d.pdf.

SECTION 1

Person-Centred Practice

CHAPTER 1

The Art of Caring Where Technology Is an Enabler

Antonia Brown

LEARNING OUTCOMES

At the end of this chapter, the nurses will be able to:
- Consider the art of nursing and midwifery as a concept, and place that in the context of a technology enabled world.
- Explore misconceptions around remote monitoring and what it means for nursing and midwifery.
- Consider the implications of digitally native generations for nursing and midwifery practice.
- Examine required skills for retention of the art of nursing and midwifery in the modern age.

Introduction

Throughout its history, nursing and midwifery practice has been described as an art and a science. Florence Nightingale was one of the first to talk about nursing and midwifery as an art, when she described how the profession was more than just technical and administrative tasks, and was more about understanding individual patient needs (Nightingale, 1860). As of 2023, it could be said that the science has overtaken the art, with more pressure on nurses and midwives to look after patients in greater numbers and with increasing complexity of multiple health and social care needs. Nurses and midwives are forced to rush through tasks as demand outweighs capacity, and their ability to assess conditions holistically and spend time building relationships with people is often lost.

It might be assumed technology is an enabler of the science of practice. However, this chapter outlines how technology can enable nurses to reconnect with the art of nursing and midwifery. Bailey et al. (2009) describe the artful nurse as one who knows their patient, and who is able to build reciprocity in their relationship. In the modern age, we are faced with a population that is engaged with technology. Many of them are digital natives. If nurses and midwives are to build reciprocity with these people and communities, they must engage with technology themselves. Chinn et al. (2011) talked about the art of nursing as the ability to make sense of any situation experienced by the patient, understand what needs to be done, and act on their behalf. This could apply equally to midwifery. Some groups of patients may

3

have such complex needs that the nurses and midwives may be unable to understand them without the use of complex data.

As delivering some elements of care remotely or using technology due to the dwindling numbers of nurses, midwives and other healthcare professionals becomes an increasing necessity, we also consider how the art of nursing and midwifery can be retained under circumstances where nurses are not at the bedside, or where the bedside is the bedside is a technologically dense environement.

NURSING AND MIDWIFERY INSTINCT AND COMPASSIONATE CARE

'The unique role of the nurse can never be substituted by any kind of machinery, be it a computer or otherwise. The nurse should treat them as useful tools, never as a replacement for her art' (Mann, 1992). Even in 1983, nurses were recognising that technology could offer useful tools, but that these would not replace the art of nursing and midwifery, and that ensuring this was in the hands of the practitioner themselves.

Henry (2018) said, 'the artful experience includes connecting with patients and intuitive care giving'. One of the great benefits of technology is that it connects people, bringing them together across great distances and offering opportunities to be together virtually when other barriers prevent physical meetings. Whatever the driver, whether the desire to reduce carbon footprint of the health services, a diminishing workforce leaving us shorthanded, adverse weather conditions preventing nurses from getting to a patient, or the need to reduce the risk of spreading infection, having a way to overcome that barrier and maintain connection enables implementing the art of nursing and midwifery. If technologies, such as virtual consultations, can be used to maintain connections, compassionate delivery of care is possible, just as it is in person. We have all experienced rude and unpleasant telephone calls and, conversely, have had tender and caring conversations over the phone – the technology used is just the enabler, and the potential for compassion remains with the nurses and midwives through the way they communicate.

> 'This image of socially and affectively deprived lonely persons living amongst cold and instrumental technologies … skips the fact that people do indeed develop affective relations with technologies, and that technologies may help to develop social ties rather than cutting them. A straightforward example is the mobile phone. That some people particularly love their mobile phone is hard to overlook when one sees the care with which these devices are "dressed up" and personalised. Apart from the love of the actual device, there is affection because of its functionality. The mobile phone allows its user to communicate with, stay in touch and care for other persons in many places and almost all the time. So the affection for the device may well stem from the combination of its material attractiveness and the relations that it allows for'.
>
> (Pols and Moser, 2009)

With technology becoming more adept at undertaking tasks previously carried out by people, we can imagine a future in which significant nursing and midwifery time is saved by using digital technologies. In this future, it would be sensible to consider what the role of nurses and midwives might be when some of the traditional tasks can be safely carried out by robots and artificial intelligence. With some of the tasks taken over, there might be an opportunity for 'patient interaction … getting to know more about the patient's condition, preferences, establishing an emotional connection with patients and responding appropriately to their needs … The caring aspect of nursing will be made real' (Pepito et al., 2019).

'One of the primary reasons why artificially intelligent machines seem to threaten the nursing and midwifery profession is the possibility that it would outperform human thinking. However, these machines cannot truly outperform human thinking because performance includes the subjective, constantly changing, and particularly individual nature of most scenarios. Today, an area where artificial intelligence fails to compete is in the learning process wherein individuals are continually taking in new information and expanding their personal databases. This is because artificial intelligence cannot independently form new context and learn like human beings, rather they are inherently "human-dependent". Because of this, what would likely happen is the combination of optimal human power and artificial intelligence. Combining advanced analytics of artificial intelligence with the experience, knowledge, and critical thinking skills of nurses would result in making better clinical reasoning and clinical decision-making which improves patient care at lower cost'.

(Pepito et al., 2019)

NOT WHETHER WE CAN, WHETHER WE SHOULD

It has been generally accepted in nursing and midwifery that the application of science to the care and treatment of people is necessary to provide complete care. Nurses and midwives are in the business of providing the best care they can for the benefit of people and communities, using whatever tools they have at their disposal. If we accept this, then we must also accept that technology, itself a science, may be beneficial and they must adapt their practices and develop their knowledge to provide this benefit. Nurses and midwives have a role of maximising the advantages and minimising the disadvantages of technology for people in their care (Dean, 1998). Rubeis (2021) suggests that the idea of nurses cushioning patients from the dehumanising effects of technology as 'guardians of humanity' does not go far enough; instead, nurses need to be involved in the design of technology and policymaking to ensure the person-centredness is built in.

In acute environments, technology plays a part in the care of a patient – a plethora of machines, pumps and wires surround patients in intensive care units, which are accepted as fundamental to keeping these patients alive. Within these environments, it is the nurses who maintain humanity for patients (Dean, 1998). A qualitative evidence synthesis of critical care nurses' experiences providing care for adults in highly technical environments found that while technology can pull focus away from patients, this is more common in nurses who are less familiar with the technology, than those who are familiar with it (Crilly et al., 2019). This suggests that as they get more familiar with technology, nurses and midwives will find it easier to maintain the art of nursing and midwifery while using technology to support care.

As with any other element of nursing and midwifery, experience brings proficiency, allowing the delivery of better care. As an analogy, using a needle to deliver medication is not considered a barrier to the clinician–patient relationship, because it is a necessary part of delivering treatment, even though a new nurse may find administering the injection more challenging; they may need to concentrate harder on the task and neglect conversing with the patient more than an experienced nurse, while performing the task. This is the same case with use of technology.

Given the inevitability of the digital revolution in healthcare, and the positives it can bring to people and populations when applied appropriately, it would be wise for nurses and midwives to consider where they fit in a future where digital revolution in healthcare has occurred. There is a role for clinicians in deciding whether remote monitoring or virtual care should be happening, as opposed to whether it can, or what is possible. Clinicians will be advocates for people, and for individualised care planning with consideration of appropriateness for the individual. It is clear that there must be roles for nurses and midwives 'in technology … to ensure that healthcare would fit the needs of patients' (Pepito et al., 2019).

LEARNING EXERCISE

Can you think of any examples where technology is being implemented in your workplace? Have nurses or midwives been included in the implementation? Write a list of considerations which you think should be taken into account for the implementation of technology, and how you think it could be addressed.

REMOTE AND TECHNOLOGICALLY ENABLED CARE

When thinking about care being delivered with technology as an enabler, it is difficult to not think of virtual wards and remote monitoring. Most National Health Service (NHS) Trusts in the UK are at some point on the journey of implementing virtual wards, under a directive from NHS England (NHS England, n.d.). For most patients on a virtual ward, this will involve at least some element of virtual care, which may include remote monitoring or virtual consultations. Thus, nurses will need to get used to delivering care further away from the patient bedside. As we go on this accelerated journey, with increasing numbers of virtual beds mandated every month, how can we ensure the art of nursing and midwifery remains central?

First, we must address the misconception that remote monitoring is merely monitoring of alerts and sitting in front of a computer. Skilled clinicians can use the person's data dashboards in the same way they would use paper observation charts, to identify trends and find early warnings of deterioration. They can use this information to support their decision making about whether visits are necessary. Additionally, they can supplement remotely obtained data with conversations with people or carers, alongside visits to the person if required. All of this requires clinical judgement, instinct and an understanding of the individual. The dashboards and alerts, again, are simply enablers.

Second, we need to address the fear that physical distance will mean increased risk and lack of connection. As mentioned earlier in the chapter, technology such as remote monitoring and virtual consultations are an additional means by which nurses, midwives and other clinicians can connect with people. These kinds of technology offer additional transformational opportunities to be present with persons receiving nursing and midwifery care, as they are aware of the words, silences and movements that do and do not exist (Carroll, 2018). Two principles should be kept in mind when using telehealth, which can help maintain the art of nursing and midwifery – presence (Tuxbury, 2013) and personalisation (Heckemann et al., 2016).

Lastly, we must acknowledge that remote monitoring can release more time for care; for example, in acute settings, nurses are offered the chance to speak one on one with the patient where usually they would be in a ward setting with multiple tasks to attend to. In such monitoring, travel time is reduced and remote monitoring can enable better triage, enabling them to give more time to people who have the greatest need. In a health economy, where clinicians are in short supply, anything that can give them save them some time is good for them and for the people receiving care.

DIGITAL NATIVES – A RECIPROCITY OF RELATIONSHIP

People born in and after 1980 can be defined as 'digital natives', because they have been born into a world where they are surrounded by computers, digital devices, the internet and social media. They are generally 'comfortable with and fluent in the use of technology' (Gillis, 2020). At the time of writing, the oldest digital natives are in their early 40. This group represents a large proportion of patients. People in this group are used to the convenience of banking, shopping and working online and have high expectations of healthcare being able to deliver a similar level of convenience, alongside competent, compassionate care. As Booth et al., (2021) state, 'patients are increasingly empowered, connected to the internet, and demanding personalized or self-management healthcare models that fit their busy and varied lifestyles'. Nurses and midwives are well placed to develop services with this convenience in mind, making use of digital tools to ensure that people have access to healthcare in a convenient way – perhaps 'convenience' should be added to the 6 Cs of nursing and midwifery (NHS Professionals, n.d.)!

Studies have shown that digital natives may not be convinced of the benefits of digitising healthcare (Cowey et al., 2018), perhaps because of their experience where technology was poorly implemented. For example, one participant in Cowey and Pott's study (2018) talked about preferring paper for medical documents because they can be sure of finding them again – this suggests some challenge in accessing digital documents, which could clearly be improved through more trusted systems which work every time. Technical challenges were also cited in a systematic review conducted by Leonardsen et al. (2020), with examples of faulty devices and slow connectivity leading to frustration. Digital natives have high expectations for technology to be perceived as beneficial in the delivery of healthcare.

LEARNING EXERCISE

What are some of the technologies you use every day? Think about what the important features are of these technologies which make you use them daily. How might these qualities apply to healthcare technologies?

THE ART OF NURSING AND MIDWIFERY AS AN ENABLER FOR DIGITAL TECHNOLOGY

Until now, this chapter discussed how technology can be an enabler for the art of nursing and midwifery. However, the opposite can also be true – the art of nursing and midwifery can be an enabler of technology. LeVasseur (2002) spoke about how the art of nursing and midwifery occurs when professionals gain trust to help people navigate through a challenging time. In healthcare, particularly in digital healthcare, 'trust … depends on the interplay of a complex set of enablers and impediments' (Adjekum et al., 2018). With the great many challenges associated with digital health, and distrust rife when it comes to data sharing and digital technology, there is an opportunity for nurses and midwives to use their trusted relationships with people in their care, to advocate for them, maintain trust and ensure they get the best out of digital health.

CASE STUDY

In Sussex, nurses in the children's community continence service noticed an opportunity to use digital tools to improve the experience of the children in their care. The children and their families were required to complete an array of bladder and bowel diaries and other documents before being accepted to the service, as part of the referral, and were provided with leaflets containing useful information. The service then needed to laboriously add all this information to the electronic patient record. The children and their parents were mostly digital natives, with smartphones and an expectation of digitally delivered services. The team developed an app which the families could download to input all the data, which would be shared directly with the service and negate the need for multiple forms. This app enhanced the ability of the clinicians to communicate with their patients and families, a group of digital natives, thereby supporting the art of nursing.

Conclusion

In a technology-enabled world, where numerous people are well used to the benefits of digital technologies, users are also becoming wiser to some of the risks. As nursing and midwifery professionals, we ask important questions about where our profession sits in this new world, and how we can ensure that our patients, families and communities are well served by technology, while keeping risks to a minimum. Technology is developing rapidly, irrespective of our opinion of it. Given the benefits it can bring, we would be doing our profession and the people we care for a disservice by not engaging with it. We must ensure that our voices are heard in this conversation. As nurses and midwives, we must look to the future, ensuring that we lead the way in adapting to a technologically enabled world, maintaining both our science and our art.

Key Points

1. Where the artful nurse is considered as one who is connected to people and communities, technology has a great opportunity to advance the art of nursing and midwifery by creating additional channels of communication.
2. Nurses and midwives should ensure that various routes of communication are used confidently and appropriately to enhance experience and safety.
3. Technology can present opportunities to save time for nurses and midwives, creating space for them to use their critical thinking skills, interact with patients, develop emotional connection and care, all of which are parts of the art of nursing and midwifery. Nurses and midwives should seek and ensure opportunities to maintain interaction wherever technology is employed.
4. Digital technology provides many opportunities to improve care when applied appropriately. Nurses and midwives have an opportunity to evolve their role, advocating for people and communities and helping determine when technology should and should not be deployed.
5. While technology has been seen as a communication barrier in some cases, it becomes less of a challenge as nurses and midwives become more adept at using technology. Nurses and midwives should work towards becoming proficient with technologies relevant to their clinical area, so they can use it for their patient's benefit without being distracted by it.
6. As a growing number of the population are now digital natives, and have high expectations of technology and convenience, nurses and midwives must embrace new ways of working with technology, keep pace with the populations they serve and maintain reciprocity of relationships.

References

Adjekum, A., Blasimme, A., Vayena, E., 2018. Elements of trust in digital health systems: scoping review. J. Med. Internet Res. 20 (12), e11254. https://doi.org/10.2196/11254.
Bailey, M.E., Moran, S., Graham, M.M., 2009. Creating a spiritual tapestry: nurses' experiences of delivering spiritual care to patients in an Irish hospice. Int. J. Palliat. Nurs. 15 (1), 42–48. https://doi.org/10.12968/ijpn.2009.15.1.37952.
Booth, R.G., Strudwick, G., McBride, S., et al., 2021. How the nursing and midwifery profession should adapt for a digital future. BMJ. 373, n1190. https://doi.org/10.1136/bmj.n1190.
Carroll, K., 2018. Transforming the art of nursing and midwifery: telehealth technologies. Nurs. Sci. Q. 31 (3), 230–232. https://doi.org/10.1177/0894318418774930.
Chinn, P.L., Kramer, M.K., 2011. Integrated Theory and Knowledge Development in Nursing. Mosby Elsevier, Saint Louis, MO.

Cowey, A.E., Potts, H.W.W., 2018. What can we learn from second generation digital natives? A qualitative study of undergraduates' views of digital health at one London university. Digit. Health. 4. https://doi.org/10.1177/2055207618788156.

Crilly, G., Dowling, M., Delaunois, I., et al., 2019. Critical care nurses' experiences of providing care for adults in a highly technological environment: a qualitative evidence synthesis. J. Clin. Nurs. 28 (23–24), 4250–4263. https://doi.org/10.1111/jocn.15043.

Dean, B., 1998. Reflections on technology: increasing the science but diminishing the art of nursing and midwifery? Accid. Emerg. Nurs. 6 (4), 200–206. https://doi.org/10.1016/S0965-2302(98)90080-7.

Gillis, A., 2020. What is digital native? – Definition from WhatIs.Com. Available at: https://www.techtarget.com/whatis/definition/digital-native.

Heckemann, B., Wolf, A., Ali, L., et al., 2016. Discovering untapped relationship potential with patients in telehealth: a qualitative interview study. BMJ Open. 6, e009750. https://doi.org/10.1136/bmjopen-2015-009750.

Henry D. (2018) Rediscovering the art of nursing to enhance nursing practice. Nursing Science Quarterly 31(1):47 – 54. https://doi.org/10.1177/0894318417741117.

Leonardsen, A.C.L., Hardeland, C., Helgesen, A.K., et al., 2020. Patient experiences with technology enabled care across healthcare settings – a systematic review. BMC Health Serv. Res. 20, 779. https://doi.org/10.1186/s12913-020-05633-4.

LeVasseur, J., 2002. A phenomenological study of the art of nursing: experiencing the turn. Adv. Nurs. Sci. 24 (4), 14–26.

Mann, R.E., 1992. Preserving humanity in an age of technology. Intensive Crit. Care Nurs. 8 (1), 54–59. https://doi.org/10.1016/0964-3397(92)90010-h.

NHS England. (n.d.) Virtual wards. Available at: https://www.england.nhs.uk/virtual-wards/.

NHS Professionals. (n.d.) The 6 Cs of care. Available at: https://rg-sitecore-prd-173860-cd.azurewebsites.net/nhs-staffing-pool-hub/working-in-healthcare/the-6-cs-of-care.

Nightingale, F., 1860. Notes on nursing and midwifery: what it is, and what it is not. D. Appleton and Company, New York, NY.

Pepito, J.A., Locsin, R., 2019. Can nurses remain relevant in a technologically advanced future? Int. J. Nurs. Sci. 6 (1), 106–110. https://doi.org/10.1016/j.ijnss.2018.09.013.

Pols, J., Moser, I., 2009. Cold technologies versus warm care? On affective and social relations with and through care technologies. Alter 3. (2), 159–178. https://doi.org/10.1016/j.alter.2009.01.003.

Rubeis, G., 2021. Guardians of humanity? The challenges of nursing and midwifery practice in the digital age. Nurs. Philos. 22 (2), e12331. https://doi.org/10.1111/nup.12331.

Tuxbury, J.S., 2013. The experience of presence among telehealth nurses. J. Nurs. Res. 21 (3), 155–161. https://doi.org/10.1097/jnr.0b013e3182a0b028.

CHAPTER 2

People Taking Control of Their Own Health Information

Gillian Strudwick

LEARNING OUTCOMES

At the end of this chapter, the nurses will be able to:

- Identify common technologies (e.g. patient portals) that support people in taking control of their own health information.
- Understand barriers/facilitators to the use of technologies that support people in taking control of their own health information.
- Appreciate future trends in digital healthcare delivery that support people taking control of their own health information and a more active role in their care delivery.

Introduction

There is a growing trend in healthcare contexts of individuals wanting to have better access to their health information, an increasing amount of control over who has access to it and how it is used. In general, access to all sorts of information, inclusive of health information, is easily available often at an individual's fingertips through a quick internet search. People are now able to conduct banking online, purchase their groceries, and access all sorts of services that make their lives more convenient. No wonder there is a growing expectation that technologies will support such quick access to health-related data as well.

This chapter focuses on the current and future state of people taking more control over their health information in a way that is facilitated by the use of technology. Nurses and midwives are already taking a significant leadership role in this space, advancing this agenda in healthcare. As an example, nurses are often the leads of projects and initiatives that involve making this a reality in a given organisation. In the future, nurses and midwives will have an increasingly important role in not only advocating and advancing access of health information to patients but also in identifying and providing supports to allow this to happen in both a meaningful and helpful way. The chapter begins with an overview of some of the current technologies that individuals use to obtain access to their health information. It then discusses some of the barriers to, and facilitators of, access and use of these technologies. Finally, the chapter concludes with a focus on the future, where trends and future outlooks related to increasing access to health information are described. Providing individuals with access to their data can potentially shift the power dynamic from that typically held by the nurse or midwife, to the individuals receiving care themselves. In an era of person-centred care, providing individuals with both access to and control over their health information is essential; however, doing so in a way that is helpful is still very much in a nascent stage in much of the world.

Common Technologies in Providing Individuals With Access to Their Health Information

In many (if not most) jurisdictions around the world, individuals have had the right to access their medical records for a number of years now. This is not necessarily common knowledge among healthcare consumers. Thus, for the most part, most individuals have not asked nor have had access to this information in a straightforward manner. In many hospital environments, there are departments (often called 'health records' departments) that have developed a process in which patients of that organisation can make a formal request to access their information and have it walked through with a person who understands medical jargon and helps them navigate the health record itself. Often, organisations charge money if a photocopy or printing is required. This same process is present regardless of whether the information is available in a paper or an electronic form.

In recent years, there has been a growing movement to increase individuals' access to their health records through a movement called 'OpenNotes' (OpenNotes n.d.). This movement has leveraged the current trend in healthcare of completing clinical documentation electronically, which many organisations have switched to around the world. Theoretically, electronic documentation and health records provide individuals an opportunity to digitally access their health information. In these cases, a simple login process for all individuals who receive care at an organisation can potentially negate having to go through a formal process of obtaining health records through a specific department, and encourage more individuals to access this information. Making health records available to individuals through digital means have resulted in a number of benefits. These include improved accuracy of the notes, improved adherence to medications, stronger and improved relationships between providers and patients or service users, and an enhanced ability to relay important health information to care partners (e.g. family members) (OpenNotes n.d.).

In the era of the Covid-19 pandemic, many organisations launched a patient portal, a technology that makes available health information to individuals, patients, and/or service users as quickly as possible in a digital format. These patient portals can usually be accessed through various technological devices that people use every day, such as computers, tablets and smartphones. The motivator for the launch of a patient portal by an organisation in the last several years was to be able to quickly communicate Covid-19 test results to individuals in a manner that did not strain healthcare resources. Legislation in some parts of the world has also acted as an accelerator to the adoption of this technology (U.S. Food and Drug Administration 2020). Finally, and perhaps most importantly, individuals are asking for increasing access to their health information through a digital means (like a portal), since it has become commonplace in many other aspects of their lives (e.g. banking, transportation and shopping) (Leung et al. 2019).

A patient portal is typically a secure online platform that provides individuals access to their health records (or parts of it) at a particular health organisation. This could be lab information, the results of a test, or notes written by nurses, midwives and other health professionals. There are often other functions of the patient portal as well, including appointment booking, updating contact information and completing self-assessments. Numerous organisations had patient portals prior to the pandemic; however, due to the pandemic, there has been an uptake in both availability and awareness of these by individuals.

The technology and processes described above apply to health information that is created at a health organisation by medical providers, like nurses, midwives, physicians and other health professionals. This, of course, is now understood to be just a portion of the health information that exists today. Individuals collect information about their health in other forms, for instance, through fitness applications, glucometers used in home settings, wearable heart rate monitors and mood trackers among others. This information is often held by individuals themselves, and is not accessible to healthcare providers. Nevertheless, in some cases, it may be accessible to the company or organisation which developed or sold the medical device.

LEARNING EXERCISE

You are a nurse/midwife working in a community care setting. The organisation in which you work has identified that they would like to develop a digital technology to enable patients to access their medical information, following the request of patients. You are asked to provide your feedback on what options may be feasible in your setting. What feedback do you provide? Why did you provide these suggestions?

Barriers to and Facilitators of Common Technologies That Allow Individuals to Access Their Health Information

While there are a number of potential benefits to using technology to enable individuals to access and take control over their own information, there are a number of barriers to, and facilitators of, technology use. When the concept of OpenNotes was initially introduced, there was outcry from a number of medical provider groups over concerns about individuals' access to their medical records and the notes they had written (Strudwick et al. 2018). This is despite individuals having the right to access their medical records for decades in many countries. Specifically, medical providers were concerned that their notes might not be understood, that they would receive many questions, answering which would consume their time, and that certain sensitive information could be triggering, particularly on topics such as mental illness (Strudwick et al. 2018). This concern by healthcare providers has largely been a barrier to the implementation and use of opening up clinical notes in a number of settings. However, research has explored the experiences of medical providers before and after implementing an electronic system that provides patients with access to their medical information, and found that these concerns have not been realised (Pettersson and Erlingsdóttir 2018). Thus, a potential facilitator is the supporting literature on this topic.

Other potential barriers and facilitators centre around the person accessing their health information. Both digital and health literacy are required to access medical information, since individuals typically need to login through an electronic portal, open certain health information, and interpret this information in a way that is meaningful to them. Not all individuals possess this knowledge and skillset equally to be able to do this effectively. Nurses and midwives are well positioned to support the assessments of these skills, direct individuals to reliable services and support them when gaps in this knowledge and skills are present.

There are other barriers to and facilitators of technology that enable access to an individual's personal health information. Many of these exist in the equity sphere. Accessing health information via technology assumes access to specific technological devices (e.g. tablet, smartphone and computer). It also assumes a number of other conditions that allow for this information to be viewed, such as owning or having private access to the technology, having data or reliable internet access, having the financial means to obtain the technology and on-going costs associated with using it, and having a private space to view the information. Though many people have access to relevant technologies, this is not the case for everyone. There are certain equity seeking groups that may need special support or alternative modes of providing access to health information (Crawford and Serhal 2020). For example, in rural and remote parts of Canada, high-speed internet or data/smartphone access to the internet is rarely available. Thus, certain forms of access (e.g. patient portals) may not be the most appropriate in these areas.

LEARNING EXERCISE

This learning exercise continues from the first learning exercise. The organisation you work for has decided to implement a patient portal that provides patients with access to the notes their providers have written about their care, as well as appointment booking features and access to lab results. As a nurse or midwife familiar with the potential challenges your patients might face in accessing or using the patient portal, what advice do you recommend to your organisation to enhance the adoption and use of this technology by patients?

Future Trends

To date, there has been much focus on providing curated traditional medical information in the form of documentation, clinical notes, test results and laboratory information from nurses and midwives to individuals through an electronic patient portal. This information is typically housed at the organisation in which an individual receives clinical assessments and care, be it in the community, primary care office, hospital or other settings. There is an increasing recognition that not all health information about a person may be kept in one place or at one organisation. For example, if a person goes to one organisation to receive one type of care (e.g. optometry), and then to another organisation to receive another type of care (e.g. podiatry), their health information is not consistently shared between these two providers. Currently, there is an increasing trend that will be realised in the future of improving the interoperability of the systems used by various organisations to facilitate the sharing of health information. As a part of this, individuals will need to consent to who has access to what forms of their information, and if it can be used for other purposes (e.g. research studies). Individuals should increasingly have access to their health information as this work progresses.

This discussion, however, relates to only a portion of the health-related data that likely exists, which is the medical record data. The present-day discussion is still quite centred around the providers and organisations that deliver care, and not on patient and person generated health related data. Nurses and midwives can be part of pushing this conversation forward in making it more an individual-centred focused discussion. Accordingly, individuals would need to be extensively engaged in all related decision-making processes.

One future trend is that various forms of health information that are not typically collected in medical records (e.g. fitness apps and glucometer use at home) will also be acknowledged as a part of health information that can and should be controlled by an individual. This includes acknowledging that developers, companies and those that sell consumer-focused health devices that collect data be transparent about who has access to their health data and for what purpose. In the future, it is expected that there will be increasing pressure on these developers and companies to allow individuals to make decisions about data access and control. Thus, the future of taking control of one's health information will be a context in which technology better supports individuals in being able to make decisions about what healthcare data is present, and who has access to it.

LEARNING EXERCISE

This learning exercise builds off of the previous two described in this chapter. A patient portal has been implemented in your community care organisation. Numerous patients, nurses and midwives have been consulted in the planning and implementation of the technology. Various strategies were developed to address potential barriers to the uptake and use of the patient portal, which have been successful. A recent patient satisfaction survey indicated that patients continue to want increasing access and control of their health information, as well as the opportunity to add health information from their personal devices and wearables (e.g. home monitors). As a result, the organisation is beginning to develop a road map to plan what is to come in the next 5 years with regards to providing patients with access to their own health information. You are asked to provide suggestions, ideas and comments on this matter. What do you bring forward, and why?

CASE STUDY

In Canada, a model of nursing care called 'eShift' was launched in the home and community care context. This model of nursing care emphasises people taking control over their health information and their health situation in their last remaining weeks of life. 'eShift' is a palliative care program where a single nurse remotely monitors several patients overnight, such that they can die in their own homes. They do so by being able to monitor and provide direction and oversight to non-registered care providers and family members present at home with the patient. A smartphone application is used to facilitate this process, which allows for information to be shared easily with patients and their family members in real time. This model of nursing care in the home and community care context emphasises placing patient's needs, wishes and desires for their end of life care at the centre of care. The use of technology, along with specialty trained non-registered care staff, allows nurses the opportunity to provide care to a greater number of individuals. This optimisation of nursing time is important in the current health human resource context, where there is an extreme shortage of nurses in Canada. More information about the 'eShift' model can be found here: http://healthcareathome.ca/southwest/en/Getting-Care/Getting-Care-at-Home/eshift.

Conclusion

This chapter presented an introduction to the current state and future trends in providing individuals with increasing access to their own health information through technological means. The various technologies that facilitate access to these technologies were reviewed, along with barriers to and facilitators of their use. In conclusion, nurses and midwives have played a critical role, and will continue to do so, in providing individuals with increasing access to their health information via digital technologies, as well as in supporting individuals to maximizing their use of this information. This role includes nurses and midwives being at key decision-making tables about health information management, and advocating for the inclusion of the voice and views of the patients, service users, and other individuals. The role of nurses and midwives is also to bring an equity lens to these discussions such that no individuals or groups are inadvertently left out, or behind. In addition, nurses and midwives are key players in ensuring that individuals have access to appropriate guidance, education and credible resources to guide their use and uptake of their health information through digital means. This area will continue to grow and evolve in the coming years, and nurses and midwives are well positioned to be leaders in this space.

Key Points

1. Nurses and midwives are well positioned to provide leadership in furthering the agenda of individuals having access to their own health information via digital means.
2. Various technologies already exist and are used to a variable extent throughout the world to provide patients with access to their own health information. Uptake and implementation of these current technologies could be improved.
3. In many jurisdictions around the world, people have the right to access their health information. The use of technology can facilitate access to this information in a quicker, more accessible way.
4. There are numerous barriers that currently influence the uptake of technologies that support access to health information. Nurses and midwives play a key role in identifying and implementing solutions to address these barriers.
5. Access for individuals to health information via technology will continue to grow in the future.

Technology Glossary

Digital literacy: An individual's knowledge, understanding and comfort in using digital technologies.

Electronic documentation: Clinician notes that are written in an electronic system.

Glucometer: A medical device that helps determine the blood glucose of an individual.

Interoperability: The technical connection between digital systems that allows a two-way flow of information.

OpenNotes: The concept of patients having access to the notes that their clinicians write about them.

Patient portal: A website where patients can login to view their health information.

Smartphone application: A software program designed to run on cell phones.

Wearable: A device that can be worn and tracks certain physiological parameters.

References

Crawford, A., Serhal, E., 2020. Digital health equity and COVID-19: the innovation curve cannot reinforce the social gradient of health. J. Med. Internet Res. 22 (6), e19361. https://doi.org/10.2196/19361.

Leung, K., Clark, C., Sakal, M., et al., 2019. Patient and family member readiness, needs, and perceptions of a mental health patient portal: a mixed methods study. In: Lau, F., Bartle-Clar, J.A., Bliss, G., Borycki, F. M., Courtney, K.L., Kuo, A.M.-H., Kushniruk, A., Monkman, H., Roudsari, A.V. (Eds.), Improving Usability, Safety and Patient Outcomes with Health Information Technology. IOS Press, pp. 266–270.

OpenNotes (n.d.). Let's get everyone on the same page. Available at: https://www.opennotes.org/.

Petersson, L., Erlingsdóttir, G., 2018. Open notes in Swedish psychiatric care (part 2): survey among psychiatric care professionals. JMIR Ment. Health 5 (2), 10521. https://doi.org/10.2196/10521.

Strudwick, G., Clark, C., Sanches, M., et al., 2018. Predictors of mental health professionals' perceptions of patient portals. AMIA Annu. Symp. Proc. 989–997. Available at: https://www.ncbi.nlm.nih.gov/pmc/articles/PMC6371312/.

U.S. Food and Drug Administration, 2020. 21st Century Cures Act. Available at: https://www.fda.gov/regulatory-information/selected-amendments-fdc-act/21st-century-cures-act.

Further reading

1. Irizarry, T., DeVito Dabbs, A., Curran, C.R., 2015. Patient portals and patient engagement: a state of the science review. *J. Med. Internet Res.* 17 (6), e148. https://doi.org/10.2196/jmir.4255.
2. Hodges, B.D., Paech, G., Bennett, J., 2020. Without compassion, there is no healthcare: leading with care in a technological age. McGill-Queen's University Press, Montreal.
3. Lupton, D., 2014. The commodification of patient opinion: the digital patient experience economy in the age of big data. *Sociol Health Illn.* 36 (6), 856–869. https://doi.org/10.1111/1467-9566.12109.
4. OpenNotes: https://www.opennotes.org/.

CHAPTER 3

Ensuring Digital Inclusion

Vanessa Heaslip ■ Debbie Holley

LEARNING OUTCOMES

At the end of this chapter, the nurses will be able to:
- Recognise links between determinants of health and digitalisation across people's life course.
- Have critical awareness of the range of barriers experienced by different groups regarding digital technology.
- Consider aspects of inclusive digital practice that can be taken forward into clinical roles.

Introduction

This chapter provides an overview of the principles of inclusion, and covers key terminologies, such as differences between equality and equity. It notes the global policies driving digital healthcare, recognising the potential benefits in terms of health access and quality of care. However, it also notes that unless effectively managed, digital healthcare has the potential to widen the health divide for some groups who are at risk of poorer health outcomes. Three case studies are presented as examples of those who can be digitally excluded: those experiencing homelessness; Gypsy, Roma and Travellers; and older people. Lastly, it introduces the notion that nurses and midwives play a key role in ensuring that no-one is left behind. The study provides an example of a case study where digital inclusivity is considered. Learning exercises are embedded throughout to enable nurses and midwives to see how they, in their advocacy role, can champion digital inclusion for all.

Genomics, artificial intelligence, digital medicine and robotics are all predicted to ensure safer, more productive and effective personal care for patients. The advent of telemedicine has been accelerated by the pandemic (Juniper Research 2021), and technology and digitalisation are significantly improving the experience of, and access to, healthcare professionals. Yet, assumptions of universal access underpin many such initiatives. We argue that it is important to consider these initiatives critically from an equity lens to ensure that these advancements do not widen the health divide. The terms (in)equality and (in)equity are used interchangeably. However, Heaslip et al. (2022a) argue that we need to appreciate and understand their nuanced differences to identify the challenges people can face in accessing and

TABLE 3.1 ■ Key Terms

Health inequalities	Differences that exist between groups in terms of health service access, health status and outcomes. Sometimes, inequalities are acceptable. For example, breast screening programmes for men and women are not equal.
Health equity	Achieving equity requires the provision of different attention to groups adversely affected, so equality in access, status and outcomes can be achieved.
Health inequities	Underpinned by social justice, health inequities refer to the unjust or unfair differences in health access, status and outcomes that exist between groups of people.
Health disparities	Absolute and relative differences in health status and outcomes between groups and is used to provide evidence of health inequities. For instance, differences in access to determinants of health and health services and quality of healthcare.

Source: Wilson et al. (2018).

experiencing healthcare (see Table 3.1). Digital inclusion is defined by the United Nations (UN) as 'Equitable, meaningful, and safe access to use, lead, and design of digital technologies, services, and associated opportunities for everyone, everywhere' (UN Round Table, live document).

GLOBAL POLICIES ON DIGITALISATION AND HEALTH FOR ALL

A number of global initiatives are underpinned by the desire for access to equitable health provision. Most notable are the UN Sustainable Development Goals (SDGs) set out in the 2030 Agenda for Sustainable Development as a series of aspirations, to be embodied within governmental policy agendas (United Nations 2015). Whilst we recognise that all the SDGs are related holistically in terms of the lived experiences of people across the globe, we wish to focus on the following SDGs:

- SDG 1: No poverty: end poverty in all its forms everywhere
- SDG 3: Good health and well-being: ensure healthy lives and promote well-being for all at all ages
- SDG 4: Quality education: ensure inclusive and equitable quality education and promote lifelong learning opportunities for all
- SDG 10: Reduced inequalities: within and among countries

Undoubtedly, the global Covid-19 pandemic placed a severe strain on the progress of the SDGs (United Nations 2022). Nevertheless, it also highlighted the existing global health inequities, both within and across countries, underscoring the urgent need to address these goals.

Considering the values underpinning the SDGs, the World Health Organization's (WHO) Global Strategy on Digital Health (2021) recognises that information and communication technologies present new opportunities and challenges for the achievement of these goals. The technologies can help promote health for all through the strategic and innovative use of digital technologies; however, the WHO (2021) asserts that both gender equality and health equity must be considered when planning and prioritising digital interventions to ensure that digital health technological advances do not perpetuate inequity. This commitment towards health equity and gender equality was transferred into the WHO European Regional Action Plan (WHO European Region 2022), which recognised that digital technologies must be seen as a key determinant of health (more on this later) and a main driver of health equity; consequently, member countries must develop inclusive digital societies.

Digital Exclusion

Data from the Office for National Statistics (ONS) (2019) identified that whilst the number of internet non-users has been declining in the UK, there were still 5.3 million adults or 10% of the total population, who did not use the internet, as of 2018. Of those that did use the internet, 6.4 million adults or only 12% had limited ability of using the internet. In exploring digital exclusion in higher education, Saifuddin and Mette Jun Lykkegaard (2016) identified three main contributors to digital exclusion, that we argue can be extrapolated for the general society:

- Social exclusion – low income, avoidance of technology, lack of motivation and commitment, or physical or mental disability
- Digital exclusion – lack of hardware devices and internet services
- Accessibility – division in Wi-Fi connectivity between rural and urban areas, and differences in digital and information literacy

However, other factors, including age, gender and educational attainment, are also relevant. More specifically, older people are more likely to be digitally excluded (Helsper 2017); the digital divide negatively affects women (Yang 2021); and lower education is strongly associated with non-internet use (Helsper 2017). Both Greer et al. (2019) and Helsper (2017) assert that economic disadvantage is one of the strongest determinants of digital disengagement. The Lancet and Financial Times Commission (Kickbusch et al. 2021) argued that digital transformations must be considered a new determinant of health (Fig. 3.1) due to the significant impact of digital technology on people's life course.

Considering education as an example, homeschooling during the Covid-19 pandemic negatively impacted the education of young people living in poverty due to lack of digital infrastructure in their homes (UK Parliament 2021). This can have long-term consequences for their health, as there is sufficient evidence linking school attendance and education attainment to better physical and mental health (Department of Health and Social Care 2021). Similarly, nurse education is affected by digital exclusion, despite the call for every nurse to be an 'e-nurse' by the RCN (Royal College of Nursing 2018). Indeed both the RCN and the Topal Review (2019) emphasise on the key digital skills required by nurses and midwives and the need to incorporate these into preparatory training programmes.

Nursing and midwifery programmes have seen an increased use of hybrid and online learning, simulation skills-based packages and remote working using digital

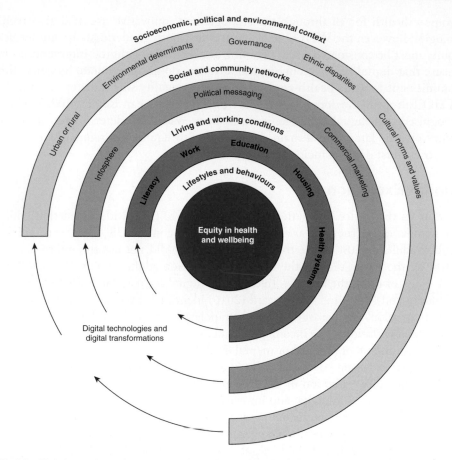

Fig. 3.1 Digital transformation as a new determinate of health (Adapted from Kickbusch et al. 2021).

technology. However, many nursing students' education is negatively affected due to poor internet connectivity (Padagas 2021). We argue that as nurse and midwifery education is committed to widening participation, by encouraging applications from young people from disadvantaged backgrounds, it would be incorrect to assume that all students have access to personal laptops. Indeed, the Office for Students' (2020) Digital Poverty report identified the compounding impact of different aspects of identity intersect which affect individuals' experiences of power and oppression in societal structures. Of particular concern was that 4% of the students reported having no internet access; this equates to 104,000 students across English Higher Education institutions with no access to the internet.

This impact of digitalisation on all aspects of people's lives and the links between digital inequity and social/societal disadvantage, Helsper (2021) argues, makes it crucial to consider socio-digital inequalities. Her Corresponding Fields model calls for a societal level exploration of the drivers of digital inequalities. These concepts have been amplified in calls for all people to become digitally literate through public and private partnerships, thus moving towards a digitally connected society (Alvarez

2021). These principles are reflected in the recently revised EU digital competence framework (Vuorikari et al. 2022). Ultimately, we must be cautious to not lay the blame on individuals and communities for their lack of digital skills, capabilities and digital linkages, as digital transformation has to be embedded within wider social, political and economic processes (Kickbusch et al. 2021).

To further explore the experiences of people who could find themselves digitally excluded, we present the following case studies: people experiencing homeless; Gypsy, Roma, Travellers and older people.

PEOPLE EXPERIENCING HOMELESSNESS

Homelessness is on the rise (European Social Policy Network 2019), and the mean age at death for people experiencing homelessness is 45.5 years for men and 43.2 years for women (ONS 2022a); as such, they are a group experiencing significant health inequity. A systematic review by Heaslip et al. (2021) identified that technology has the potential to support health and well-being of people living on the street. However, there are challenges in terms of connectivity. The review identified that mobile phone ownership ranged from 53% to 100% (including both mobile and smartphones); nevertheless, access to the internet on these devices could be poor due to limited access to Wi-Fi and poor digital literacy skills. Additionally, older people would experience more difficulties. Access to free Wi-Fi is essential for those living on the street, as they tend to rely on prepaid mobile plans, which are more expensive (Humphry 2021). Therefore, they access the internet primarily through public resources, such as libraries, internet cafés, and night shelters (Heaslip et al. 2022b), which are problematic in terms of: 1) access and 2) confidentiality when dealing with health issues. Many people experiencing homelessness also have concerns about using digital technologies, due to worries regarding who has access to their personal data (Heaslip et al. 2021); this further inhibits their use of digital technologies.

GYPSY, ROMA AND TRAVELLERS

Gypsy, Roma and Traveller communities experience significant health inequities linked to higher mortality, morbidity and infant mortality, as well as difficulties in accessing healthcare (Heaslip et al. 2019). Studies regarding digital access of these communities have produced mixed results, with some writers arguing poor (Garmendia 2019) and others noting good (Salemink 2016) access and connectivity, depending on location, site provision and country of residence. Research in the UK by Scadding and Sweeney (2018) with Gypsies and Travellers identified that 20% had never used the internet, 52% reported low confidence in using the internet and only 38% had a household internet connection; the proportion is much lower when compared to that of people living outside these communities.

Gypsy, Roma and Travellers typically use their smartphones to communicate with other people in the community or family through closed social media sites, such as WhatsApp or Facebook (Garmendia 2019; Salemink 2016). Digital literacy is low in these communities (Garmendia 2019; Salemink 2016), largely due to poor literacy skills in general (Scadding 2018); this can further inhibit wider use of digitalisation, especially for older people. Salemink (2016) argues there is a gender aspect, as women spend more time at home, thereby obtaining more opportunity to develop digital skills, compared to men who are at greater risk of digital exclusion. Reasons for low internet use was linked to age (above 40), which is much younger than those in non-Gypsy/Traveller communities, as well as challenges with connectivity due to cost of the internet (Scadding 2018). Many Gypsy, Roma and Travellers live in rural communities or travel in rural areas, which worsens the connectivity problem (Townsend et al. 2020).

OLDER PEOPLE

Unlike the two communities mentioned above, both of which experience overt discrimination and marginalisation, older people are less stigmatised; nevertheless, they can also find themselves marginalised in terms of digital exclusion. The number of older people both in the UK and globally is increasing, especially in the >80 years age group (WHO 2022). The most recent 2021 Census identified that in the UK, there are over 11 million people (18.6% of the total population) aged 65 and older, of which 527,900 are ≥90 years old (ONS 2022b). Specifically, older people are not a homogeneous group but consist of people from different ethnicities, social, economic and health status; these intersectionalities may have an impact upon their health, well-being and access to services.

Older people are at risk of digital exclusion because they are less likely to utilise communication devices, such as smartphones and tablets (Hill et al. 2015). A large multi-cohort study of 108,621 participants revealed digital exclusion in older people across countries: 23.8% (Denmark), 30.4% (England), 65.5% (Mexico) and 96.9% (China) (Lu et al. 2022). However, intersectionality is important, as Liu (2021) identified that Black and minority ethnic females with lower social status have the lowest computer and smartphone ownership. This research also showed a decline in online information seeking amongst white males, regardless of social status, and black and ethnic minority males and females with a lower social status. Digital exclusion in older people is influenced by a lack of digital literacy. Gallistl et al. (2021) identified lack of training and support as barriers to digital engagement. Furthermore, trust in using digital technology is lower in older people, compared to younger users (Mubarak 2022). There is a link between digital inclusion and health, as research identified that functional dependency increased in the digitally excluded (Lu et al. 2022).

LEARNING EXERCISE

Reflecting on excluded groups

Considering the three case studies presented previously, take one of these groups and apply it to your service. Reflect upon:
  1) how you communicate with clients from this group regarding access to services and wider resources available.
  2) how much of this communication utilises digital aspects.
  3) what barriers and challenges they may face in accessing your service.
  4) what alternative provision could be provided.

One way to promote digital inclusivity is through the use of digital intermediaries (Warren 2007). These are typically friends or family members who assist those digitally excluded and enable them to utilise digital technology (such as completing online forms and internet shopping). Whilst this is beneficial, there are issues regarding confidentiality and privacy with regards to relying on personal intermediaries. As such, we argue that any further growth in digital healthcare provision be matched by a growth in professional digital healthcare intermediaries to support those digitally excluded and help them navigate the digital resources provided. Furthermore, we assert the need for an investment in digital champions and digital training to support those who lack digital literacy.

Role of Nurses and Midwives

Despite the advances in technological and digital health, there are concerns that nurses and midwives have not kept pace with the rapid changes in digital technology (Booth et al. 2021). However, the nursing and midwifery profession is diverse; as such, they may also face challenges in accessing and utilising digital technology and therefore, find themselves digitally excluded. Indeed, research conducted by the Royal College of Nursing (2018) with 896 nurses and midwives identified that 81% perceived that data information, knowledge and technology would positively contribute to nursing and midwifery; however, less than 50% felt that their organisation was supportive in helping them develop their digital capabilities.

LEARNING EXERCISE

Map your digital skills

1) Please access one of these digital capability frameworks and undertake a self-assessment of the areas of competence.
   a. Health Education England
      https://www.hee.nhs.uk/sites/default/files/documents/Digital%20 Literacy%20Capability%20Framework%202018.pdf.
   b. The Australian Digital Literacy Self-Assessment Tool (2020)
      https://thinkspace.csu.edu.au/digitalcitizenshipguideetl523/digital-literacy-self-assessment-tool/.
2) Investigate whether your Trust has a Chief Nurse Information Officer (CNIO) and explore what your Trust is doing to improve the staff's digital inclusion.

We argue one does not need to be an expert in digital health to influence the digital agenda. Nurses or midwives have significant expertise about their service and the population they work with. As such, they have a key role in emphasising to their organisation the impact of digitalisation on their clients, including highlighting the digitally excluded groups and advocating for their ability to access all dimensions of the services (including digital). This advocacy may include being part of task and finish groups and helping develop new digital technologies to ensure it is user friendly, patient centred and inclusive.

CASE STUDY

To support readers to consider how they can build or ensure digital inclusivity, we share an example: the Greater Manchester Kidney Information Network (GMKIN), which was set up in 2013 and aims to support people living with kidney disease (Vasilica and Ormandy 2017). The network comprises three main online sites, including:

- GMKIN website (www.kinet.site), which includes informational pages, a forum, blogs and commentaries
- GM Kidney Information Network Facebook page
- Twitter @GMKInet

At the development of the network, engagement of users was recognised as essential. This was facilitated through the network development group consisting of patients/carers (n = 10) and health practitioners (n = 5), who worked together to co-design the network (Vasilica 2015). This was done in three stages. Stage 1 was an initial consultation, where different social media platforms were reviewed to explore what was good, and the potential hub was explored. Stage 2 consisted of a presentation of the hub and discussions regarding colour, usability and accessibility (creating accounts, writing and sharing posts and adding comments). Stage 3 consisted of platform testing and virtual meetings to refine the hub before it was released to the public. At Stage 3, a forum was developed on the GMKIN platform to allow patients/carers to post technical queries and support each other, thus building social support (Vasilica 2015).

Inclusivity was also built into the testing stage, as patients who were not regular internet users were recruited. They were provided with an iPad and a broadband connection which enabled them to go online. They received training from the researcher so that their feedback regarding the site could be incorporated. This training typically lasted for an hour to build confidence in using the technology, and was supplemented by step-by-step user guides (Vasilica 2015). This example demonstrates the important principles of digital inclusivity, namely co-production with people as well as consideration and amelioration of some of the barriers to digital inclusivity.

Conclusion

Digitalisation is a fundamental component of contemporary society and as such, nurses and midwives must consider it integral to the wider determinants of health across the life course. There is high possibility that digitalisation can help ensure health for all. However, to achieve this, all communities that nurses and midwives work with should be able to access and utilise any digital services that are developed. Universal access cannot be assumed and it must be recognised that many individuals and communities can find themselves digitally excluded, including nurses and midwives. Nurses and midwives have a professional responsibility to ensure that any digital health services developed consider those who experience digital exclusion. Failure to do so risks widening the health divide for individuals and communities that already experience health inequity.

Key Points

1. We must critically challenge perceptions of universal digital access, recognising that there are individuals and communities that experience digital exclusion. We must also consider the impact of intersectionality, which compounds exclusion.
2. We must critically examine our current provision, exploring whether there are aspects of our services which unintentionally exclude those experiencing digital exclusion and seek ways to address this.
3. People who are marginalised and experience discrimination may lack trust in digital healthcare technology. We as nurses and midwives must feel confident in the digital services offered, so we can build trust in their use.
4. We must be aware of digital innovation being considered within our organisations and use our advocacy role to ensure they enable inclusion for all.
5. We must ensure robust evaluation of new services in terms of equity and the degree to which they do or do not facilitate access for those digitally excluded.

References

Alvarez Jr., A.V., 2021. Rethinking the digital divide in the time of crisis. Globus J. Prog. Educ. 11 (1), 26–28.

Booth, R., Strudwick, G., McBride, S., et al., 2021. How the nursing profession should adapt for a digital future. Br. Med. J. 373, n1190. https://doi.org/10.1136/bmj.n1190.

Department of Health and Social Care, 2021. Research and Analysis: Education, Schooling and Health Summary. Available at: https://www.gov.uk/government/publications/education-schooling-and-health/education-schooling-and-health-summary.

European Social Policy Network, 2019. Fighting Homelessness and Housing Exclusion in Europe: A Study of National Policies. European Social Policy Network, Brussels, Belgium.

Gallistl, V., Rohner, R., Hengl, L., 2021. Doing digital exclusion – technology practices of older internet non-users. J. Ageing Stud. 59, 100973. https://doi.org/10.1016/j.jaging.2021.100973.

Garmendia, M., Karrera, I., 2019. ICT use and digital inclusion among Roma/Gitano adolescents. Media Commun. 7 (1), 22–31.

Greer, B., Robotham, D., Simblett, S., et al., 2019. Digital exclusion among mental health service users: qualitative investigation. J. Med. Internet Res. 21 (1), 1–9.

Heaslip, V., Green, S., Simkhada, B., et al., 2022b. How do people who are homeless find out about local health and social care services: a mixed method study. Int. J. Environ. Res. Publ. Health 19 (1), 46. https://doi.org/10.3390/ijerph19010046.

Heaslip, V., Richer, S., Simkhada, B., et al., 2021. Use of technology to promote health and wellbeing of people who are homeless: a systematic review. Int. J. Environ. Res. Publ. Health. 18 (13), 6845. https://doi.org/10.3390/ijerph18136845.

Heaslip, V., Thompson, R., Tauringana, M., et al., 2022a. Health inequity in the UK: exploring health inequality and inequity. Pract. Nurs. 33 (2), 84–87.

Heaslip, V., Wilson, D., Jackson, D., 2019. Are Gypsy, Roma, Travellers Communities Indigenous and Would Identification as Such Better Address Their Public Health Needs? Public Health. 176, 43–49. https://doi.org/10.1016/j.puhe.2019.02.020.

Helsper, E., 2021. The Digital Disconnect: The Social Causes and Consequences of Digital Inequalities. SAGE Publications Ltd, London.

Helsper, E., Reisdorf, B.C., 2017. The emergence of a 'digital underclass' in Great Britain and Sweden: changing reasons for digital exclusion. New Media Soc. 19 (8), 1253–1270.

Hill, R., Betts, L.R., Gardner, S.E., 2015. Older adults' experiences and perceptions of digital technology: (dis)empowerment, wellbeing, and inclusion. Comput. Hum. Behav. 48, 415–423.

Humphry, J., 2021. Looking for Wi-Fi: youth homelessness and mobile connectivity in the city. Inf. Commun. Ethics Soc. 24 (7), 1009–1023.

Juniper Research, 2021. The Doctor Is Always in: How Teleconsultations Improve Patient Care. Available at: https://www.juniperresearch.com/whitepapers/how-teleconsultations-improve-patient-care.

Kickbusch, I., Piselli, D., Agrawal, A., et al., 2021. The Lancet and financial times commission on governing health futures 2030 – growing up in a digital world. Lancet 398, 1727–1776.

Liu, B., 2021. The impact of intersectionality of multiple identities on digital health divide, quality of life and loneliness among older adults in the UK. Br. J. Soc. Work 51, 3077–3097.

Lu, X., Yao, Y., Jin, Y., 2022. Digital exclusion and functional dependence in older people: findings from five longitudinal cohort studies. Lancet 54, 1–11. https://doi.org/10.1016/j.eclinm.2022.101708.

Md, S., Lykkegaard P, M.J., 2016. Digital exclusion in higher education contexts: a systemic literature review. Procedia Social and Behavioural Sciences 228, 614–621.

Mubarak, F., Suomi, R., 2022. Elderly forgotten? Digital exclusion in the information age and the rising grey digital divide. Inquiry – The J. Health Care Organ. Provis. Financing 59, 1–7. https://doi.org/10.1177/00469580221096272.

Office for National Statistics (ONS), 2019. Exploring the UK's Digital divide. Available at: https://www.ons.gov.uk/peoplepopulationandcommunity/householdcharacteristics/home internetandsocialmediausage/articles/exploringtheuksdigitaldivide/2019-03-04.

Office for National Statistics (ONS), 2022a. Deaths of Homeless People in England and Wales: 2021 Registrations. Available at: https://www.ons.gov.uk/peoplepopulationandco mmunity/birthsdeathsandmarriages/deaths/bulletins/deathsofhomelesspeopleinenglanda ndwales/2021registrations.

Office for National Statistics (ONS), 2022b. Voices of Our Ageing Population: Living Longer Lives. Available at: https://www.ons.gov.uk/peoplepopulationandcommunity/b irthsdeathsandmarriages/ageing/articles/voicesofourageingpopulation/livinglongerlives #:~:text=The%20population%20of%20England%20and,the%20previous%20census%2 0in%202011.

Office for Students, 2020. Digital Poverty. Available at: https://www.officeforstudents.org.uk /news-blog-and-events/press-and-media/digital-poverty-risks-leaving-students-behind.

Padagas, R., 2021. Overcoming Digital divide: Lessons from Nursing Students with Low to Absent Connectivity and Capability. Proceedings of the 29th International Conference on Computers in Education. Asia-Pacific Society for Computers in Education. Available at: https://icce2021.apsce.net/wp-content/uploads/2021/12/ICCE2021-Vol.II-PP.-732-734.pdf.

Parliament, U.K., 2021. Covid-19: Impact on Child Poverty and on Young People's Education, Health and Wellbeing. Available at: https://lordslibrary.parliament.uk/covid-19-impact-on-child-poverty-and-on-young-peoples-education-health-and-wellbeing/#:~:text=T he%20huge%20disruption%20to%20schooling,seen%20prior%20to%20the%20pandemic.

Royal College of Nursing, 2018. Every Nurse an E-Nurse. Royal College of Nursing, London.

Salemink, K., 2016. Digital margins: social and digital exclusion of gypsy-travellers in the Netherlands. Environ. Plann. 48 (6), 1170–1187.

Scadding, J., Sweeney, S., 2018. Digital Exclusion in Gypsy and Traveller Communities in the UK. Friends Families and Travellers. Available at: https://www.gypsy-traveller.org/wp-content/uploads/2018/09/Digital-Inclusion-in-Gypsy-and-Traveller-communities-FINAL-1.pdf.

The Topal Review, 2019. Preparing the Healthcare Workforce to Deliver the Digital Future. Available at: https://topol.hee.nhs.uk/the-topol-review/#:~:text=The%20Topol%20Revie w%20outlined%20recommendations%20to%20ensure%20the,else%20in%20the%20worl d.%20About%20the%20Topol%20Review.

Townsend, L., Salemink, K., Wallace, C.D., 2020. Gypsy–Traveller communities in the United Kingdom and The Netherlands: socially and digitally excluded? Media Cult. Soc. 42 (5), 637–653. https://doi.org/10.1177/016344371880738.

United Nations, 2022. The Sustainable Development Goals Report 2022. Available at: https://unstats.un.org/sdgs/report/2022/The-Sustainable-Development-Goals-Report-2022.pdf.

United Nations (undated), Digital Inclusion. Available at: Definition_Digital-Inclusion.pdf(un.org).

United Nations Sustainable Development Goals, 2015. Resolution Adopted by the General Assembly on 25 September 2015. Available at: https://documents-dds-ny.un.org/doc/UN DOC/GEN/N15/291/89/PDF/N1529189.pdf?OpenElement.

Vasilica, C.M., 2015. Impact of Using Social media to Increase Patient Information Provision, Networking and Communication. Doctor of Philosophy; School of Nursing. Social Work and Social Science, University of Salford, Midwifery.

Vasilica, C.M., Ormandy, P., 2017. Methods for Studying Information Provision, Networking and Communication in Patient Support Groups. In: Urquhart, C., Hamad, F., Tbaishat, D., Yeoman, A. (Eds.), Information Systems: Process and Practice. Facet Publishing, London, pp. 205–233.

Vuorikari, R., Kluzer, S., Punie, Y., 2022. DigComp 2.2: The Digital Competence Framework for Citizens – with New Examples of Knowledge, Skills and Attitudes. Publication Office of the European Union, Luxembourg.

Warren, M., 2007. The digital vicious cycle: links between social disadvantage and digital exclusion in rural areas. Telecommun. Pol. 31, 374–388.

Wilson, D., Heaslip, V., Jackson, D., 2018. Improving equity and cultural responsiveness with marginalised communities: understanding competing worldviews. J. Clin. Nurs. 27 (19–20), 3810–3819. https://doi.org/10.1111/jocn.14546.

World Health Organization (WHO), 2021. Global Strategy on Digital Health 2020–2025. Available at: https://www.who.int/docs/default-source/documents/gs4dhdaa2a9f352b04 45bafbc79ca799dce4d.pdf.

World Health Organization (WHO), 2022. Ageing and Health. Available at: https://www.who.int/news-room/fact-sheets/detail/ageing-and-health.

World Health Organization European Region, 2022. Regional Digital Health Action Plan for the WHO European Region 2023–2030. Available at: https://apps.who.int/iris/bit-stream/handle/10665/360950/72wd05e-DigitalHealth-220529.pdf?sequence=2&isAllo wed=y.

Yang, J., Du, P., 2021. Gender, capital endowment and digital exclusion of older people in China. Ageing Soc. 41, 2502–2526.

SECTION 2

Leadership and a Digitally Ready Workforce

CHAPTER 4

Supporting Digital Literacy

Henrietta Mbeah ■ Cristina Vasilica

LEARNING OUTCOMES

At the end of this chapter, the nurses will be able to:
- Consider the importance of digital literacy as a core competence for nurses.
- Understand the practice and policy drivers affecting the development of digital competence for nursing.
- Critically evaluate contextual factors that facilitate or hinder the development of nurses' digital literacy.
- Consider tools and resources that can support digital literacy.
- Consider the emergence of new nursing roles for digital care.

Introduction

There is increasing recognition that the nursing workforce is critical to contributing to the maintenance of global health through their roles, education, research, leadership and service delivery (WHO 2021). The rapid development of digital technologies and use in healthcare education and training requires providing the healthcare workforce with the preparedness and skills to fully utilise the innovative technologies available to them.

Healthcare delivery has evolved along with the increasing use of digital and other innovative technologies. The benefits that technology affords us can only fully be realised with a digitally ready health workforce that has the skills and right attitude towards digital technologies. This will be required alongside contribution from technical experts (Health Education England [HEE] 2021; HEE 2019; Wachter 2016).

Thus, it is imperative that digital literacy be developed and enhanced across the workforce, especially for nursing and midwifery staff, who form nearly 50% of the health workforce, are the biggest professional group globally (WHO 2020), and spend the most time with individuals or patients receiving care (Butler et al. 2018). Development of digital skills for the nursing and midwifery workforce is required across a continuum, from pre-qualification or pre-registration to board level leadership.

Digital literacy has several definitions. However, the focus of discussions in this chapter is based on the HEE's definition: 'those capabilities that fit someone for living, learning, working, participating, and thriving in a digital society' (HEE 2018). The HEE digital capabilities framework for health and care staff underpins this definition (Fig. 4.1). The capabilities framework was an adaptation of the Joint Information Systems Committee (JISC) framework (2014). The Australian Digital

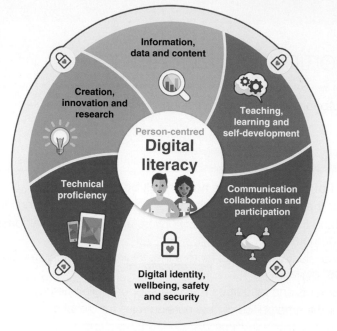

Fig. 4.1   Person-centred digital literacy. (Adapted from JISC framework 2014)

Health Agency (2020) has established a specific framework for nurses, National Nursing and Midwifery Digital Health Capability Framework.

While it is important to develop digital literacy of nurses, midwives and the wider health workforce, full utilisation of the skills acquired is dependent on other factors, such organisational culture and the availability of the appropriate technologies.

Digital Literacy for Nurses

The term digital literacy or digital literacies has been debated by various individuals and sectors over the last two decades. UNESCO (2011) described digital literacy as consisting of a set of 'basic skills' required for working with digital media, information processing and retrieval, participating in social networks for knowledge creation and dissemination, and a wide range of professional computing skills. This definition has evolved with the recognition that individuals require more than 'basic skills' to be deemed digitally literate. Recent definitions of digital literacy include 'the power to use digital tools to solve problems, produce innovative projects, enhance communication, and prepare for the challenges of an increasingly digital world' (Adobe Creative Campus EduMax 2019). This definition, and others such as those from JISC and HEE, captures the multifaceted nature of digital literacy and provides an all-encompassing definition that can be applied to different contexts, for example, work, education and everyday life.

This definition captures the multifaceted nature of digital literacy and provides an all-encompassing definition that can be applied to different contexts, for example work, education and everyday life. But what does it mean to be a digitally literate nurse? The National Nursing & Midwifery Digital Health Capability Framework (ADHA 2020) was developed in response to the need for profession specific digital capability competencies that can be used across the breadth of clinical practice. It covers five domains digital professionalism, leadership and advocacy, data and information quality, information enabled care and technology. Using a spectrum of formative to proficient It is designed to assess the digital competence of all nurses from generalist to those leading the digital health agenda. Such approaches have not been adopted globally and widespread variation in the education of nurses for digital healthcare exists. Arguably this reflects the widespread variation in digital healthcare maturity globally.

The development of digital literacy for nurses continues to be driven by individual, organisational, professional and regulatory requirements.

Professional and Policy Drivers

There are several professional, regulatory, practice and policy drivers for promoting and developing digital literacy within the workforce.

Recent evidence suggests the critical need for digital literacy for employability, economic growth and competitiveness in the labour market (OECD 2016). The health sector is always striving to improve the quality of care, improve patient or service user experience and use resources well. Additionally, the changing demands and complexity of healthcare provision, alongside increasing use of technology, have initiated the prioritisation of digital literacy to support the health workforce in performing their roles effectively.

The Nursing and Midwifery Council (NMC), UK, in their standards of proficiency for nurses (2018), expects every nurse and midwife at the point of registration to demonstrate digital and technological skills required to meet the needs of people in their care to ensure safe and effective practice. The NMC's expectation of its registrants also includes the effective and responsible use of a range of digital technologies to access, input, share and apply information and data within teams and between agencies, and finally, to analyse and clearly record and share digital information and data by applying digital literacy skills.

The strive for increased digital literacy is driven not only by healthcare regulators, such as the Nursing and Midwifery Council, and professional bodies, such as the Royal Colleges of Nursing (2018) but also by other government agencies across the globe.

Governments across the globe have been exploring effective strategies and investments to support digital literacy development of the health workforce. The UK has commissioned various reports and reviews to investigate the subject, including Wachter's (2016) report and the Topol Review (HEE 2019). These reports identified the need for greater development in digital skills across the health and social care workforce and the need to develop a digitally ready workforce, respectively.

The latest review that is expected to have tremendous implications for digital literacy and digital roles for nurses is the Philips Ives review in the UK.

CONTEXTUAL FACTORS THAT FACILITATE OR HINDER EFFECTIVE DIGITAL LITERACY DEVELOPMENT

The development of digital literacy has become centre stage in the world with investments made in varying degrees to address this need. However, there are some challenges that must be addressed to make interventions effective.

There is no consensus on the definition of digital literacy, nor is there a consistent approach to measuring it. This has resulted in the uncertainty regarding adopting the most appropriate resources, and in inconsistent approaches to measuring digital literacy levels within our workforces, including nurses.

Several challenges can impact the development of digital literacy of the workforce, including culture, lack of funding, lack of strategy, lack of commitment and impact on digital wellbeing (JISC 2014). A concern expressed by nurses is the worry that the use of technologies will dehumanise patient care. Technology has the potential to impact on the well-being of the health workforce, who have had to rapidly adopt its use, sometimes without training and preparation (European Health Policy 2020). These concerns can impact the attitude towards adopting digital technologies and developing digital literacy skills. However, evidence suggests that the effective use of technologies to manage administrative and other manual tasks can create opportunities for care (HEE 2019). This will require the right level of digital literacy, confidence, and motivation to use the technologies.

Other contextual factors that can facilitate or hinder the development of digital literacy include lack of time for learning during working hours and organisational policies.

The availability of a plethora of tools, approaches and significant amount of learning resources can positively impact the ability of nurses in identifying the most appropriate route to take on their digital literacy journey. Conversely, the desired effect will not be achieved if the direction is not provided on the suitability of the tools, with clear signposting to quality assured curated learning materials.

DEPLOYING DIGITAL LITERACY TOOLS AND RESOURCES

The use of available tools to support digital literacy assessment and interventions is varied. Research has identified many available digital literacy assessment tools and resources. This investigation also tested a prototype digital literacy tool to establish its usability and acceptability by various healthcare professionals. The investigation concluded that there was no single existing tool that can fully be adopted and used in healthcare. This finding was in addition to the participants highlighting that they will only be motivated to use digital literacy assessment tools if recommended by their peers.

The approach taken by the health sector in England is to use an interactive self-reported Digital Skills Assessment Tool, which overlays the HEE Health and Care Digital Capabilities Framework. The tool is also used by some universities in nursing education to ensure that nurses had achieved the expected levels of digital literacy at the time of graduation. Alongside the approach being adopted in England, the Australian government and the Australian Digital Health Agency are also driving the use of the National Nursing and Midwifery Digital Health Capability Framework to support nurses in obtaining the required digital skills for their role. This is a profession specific framework which is critical for developing digital literacy amongst nurses. However, the lack of interactivity and signposting to resources may impact the full utilisation of the capability framework.

CASE STUDY

The University of Salford Digital Skills Passport ('DiSk Pass™') responds to key strategies and policy by incorporating digital capabilities within pre-registration nursing training (as recommended by HEE 2019). It aims to equip all students (future healthcare workforce) with digital capabilities (functional skills, technical resilience, digital health knowledge, confidence, and values) to thrive in today's digital world, and prepare them to learn for the future. The learning content is focused on three domains: 'digital professionalism', 'harnessing the power of digital technology' and 'your digital future'. The curriculum is informed by continuous conversations with providers, patients and current research evidence on digital health. DiSK Pass has been designed to meet the NMC's realising professionalism: standards for education and training; NMC standards framework for nursing and midwifery education (NMC, 2018); as well as HEE's Digital Capabilities Framework (HEE, 2018), equipping students with level 2 competencies in digital capabilities.

The impact of DiSk Pass™ is measured by a longitudinal study that captures students' confidence, competence, and application to practice. Preliminary evidence points towards this learning solution being perceived as being 'enlightening', 'informative', 'educative', 'resourceful', 'engaging', 'feels good to be ahead' and equipping the learner with digital competencies. Students produce novel digital solutions to current challenges. Student's digital philosophies (submitted to meet the requirement of DiSk Pass™) demonstrate a shift in how technology is perceived by student nurses and a desire for continuous personal development:

> *'I believe that digital health week has inspired many students to think more deeply about the care they provide and how changes can be made to improve care and safe practice moving into the future of nursing. This has made me more excited about my future as a nurse and how I can help to develop the use of digital health'.*
>
> **Student nurse**

This indicates that focused digital capabilities training can potentially create the foundation for a digitally enabled future and a culture where digital is valued and forms an integral part of care.

IMPACT OF POOR DIGITAL LITERACY

Automation and artificial intelligence are changing the nature of, and highlighting the greatest need for obtaining, advanced level technological skills (Bughin et al. 2018; HEE 2019).

Furthermore, demand for leadership skills is expected to rise, whereas the growth for higher cognitive skills is expected be moderate overall; however, demand is expected to rise sharply for some of these skills, especially creativity (Bughin et al. 2018). This is another indication of the critical need for digital literacy skills amongst the health workforce – particularly, nurses.

According to Australian Digital Health (2020), nurses need digital capabilities to support five main activities: professionalism, leadership and advocacy, data and information quality, information enabled care and technology.

The areas identified which encompass the delivery of professional nursing and midwifery care highlight how crucial the development of digital literacy is in providing quality, safe and efficient care. A lack of digital literacy impacts the ability to adopt digital technologies (HEE 2017), which will consequently impact a nurse's ability to provide safe and quality patient care. It has already been highlighted that digital skills are critical to employability and career progression; hence, poor digital skills can impact nurses in this way (OECD 2016).

INSIGHTS INTO DIGITAL NURSING AND MIDWIFERY ROLES

Technology is advancing rapidly, with evidence of its impact on nurses' roles (HEE 2019) and digital roles becoming commonplace. The use of increasing technology. There are over thirty digital roles within the healthcare sector in England predominantly categorised under professional, managerial and leadership roles with these subcategories: Data and Information Architecture/Application, Information and Communication Technology, and Technology Supported Transformation (HEE 2021).

While there are several digital roles for nurses to pursue, the greatest need is for professionals and specialists in clinical informatics and information management, which is anticipated to grow over the next decade (HEE 2021).

There is also an expectation that digital nurse roles will grow. However, the establishment of these roles depends on capacity and capability building through clear articulation of the development of career pathways for nurses and the establishment of professional accreditation and recognition of such roles.

Other areas that are growing and could widen the digital roles of nurses include innovation, artificial intelligence and entrepreneurship. The rise in demand for entrepreneurship and initiative taking will be the fastest growing, with a 32 percent rise in Europe and a 33 percent increase in the United States (Bughin et al. 2018).

Nurses can successfully pursue various digital careers with structures and systems in place to support them, including a developed faculty that is able to educate the future workforce using various technologies, clear definition of digital careers, recognition of digital careers and specialism as part of professional registration or accreditation. It also includes career and capability frameworks to provide transparent development pathway and flexibility by employers to recognise the critical value that hybrid careers digital skills and specialism adds to care provision.

Advance practice pillars centre around research, clinical practice, leadership and management and education. For contemporary nursing and midwifery practice, digital must be a core pillar, from preregistration or pre-license period through an individual's entire career.

LEARNING EXERCISE

How many digital roles do you know? If there was an opportunity to pick one, which role would you be most interested in and would be motivated to pursue?

Conclusion

The role of nurses in contemporary healthcare has been significantly shaped by the rapid evolution of innovative technologies. It requires nurses to not only embrace their use but also develop sound digital literacy skills.

There are various individual, organisation and systemic challenges to effectively assessing and developing digital literacy skills. There are several tools and resources to develop digital literacy. For nurses, the National Nursing and Midwifery Digital Health Capability Framework (2020) is the only profession-specific digital literacy capability framework. Developing fundamental digital literacy skills is crucial to pursuing digital nurse careers.

Digitally literate educators offer opportunities to use a blend of sound and innovative pedagogical approaches to achieve the maximum benefit out of teaching and learning (JISC 2014).

The UK higher education system has a crucial role to play in developing the skills, adaptability and mindset that goes with being digitally literate and, in doing so, produce professionals for a workplace that is being rapidly transformed by technology (The Consultancy 2021).

Nurses have high prospects of successfully pursuing digital careers and will require signposting to these roles, flexibility to pursue dual roles and systemic support and recognition of the additional skills acquired or being used. This is explored further in the next chapter.

Key Points

1. The development of digital literacy is fundamental to the roles of nurses. Critical consideration should be made about when and how development should be done.
2. There are various definitions, tools and resources that can be used to establish digital literacy skills. It is crucial to understand whether an organisation is using specific tools and resources to support professionals for their digital literacy development.
3. There are several drivers to developing and using digital literacy skills, including professional and policy drivers. However, the key to effectively establishing and using digital literacy skills is an individual having the right attitude towards digital technologies, acquiring skills and confidence and having the motivation to use the established skills.
4. The nature of nurses' role can sometimes limit the opportunities to pursue learning. Thus, it is important to utilise available tools and recommended quality assured learning.
5. There are several digital roles that nurses can pursue, including engaging in various digital learning and development opportunities to determine which pathway to follow.

References

Adobe Creative Campus EduMax, 2019. Digital Literacy in Higher Education: Highlights from EduMAX 2019 5th Anniversary.

Australian Digital Health Agency, 2020. The National Nursing and Midwifery Digital Health Capability Framework. Available at: https://anmj.org.au/the-national-nursing-and-midwifery-digital-health-capability-framework-what-it-is-and-how-to-use-it/#:~:text=The%20framework%20defines%20the%20digital%20health%20knowledge%2C%20skills,across%20a%20range%20of%20digital%20health%20specific%20domains.

Bughin, J., Hazan, E., Lund, S., et al., 2018. Skill Shift Automation and the Future of the Workforce. McKinsey and Company. Available at: mgi-skill-shift-automation-and-future-of-the-workforce-may-2018.Pdf (mckinsey.com).

Butler, R., Monsalve, M., Thomas, G.W., et al., 2018. Estimating time physicians and other health care workers spend with patients in an intensive care unit using a sensor network. Am. J. Med. 131 (8), 927.e9–e15. https://doi.org/10.1016/j.amjmed.2018.03.015.

European Health Policy (EHP), 2020. EHP7 Policy Recommendations. Recover, Reinvest, Reinvent: Creating a Resilient European Health Union. Available at: https://www.healthparliament.eu/wp-content/uploads/2022/07/EHP7_Policy_Book.pdf#EHP7_Policy_Book.indd:2%20-%20Future-Proofing%20Health%20Systems:85.

Health Education England, 2017. Digital Literacy: Existing Educational Resource Mapping and Analysis. Health Education England, London.

Health Education England, 2018. A Health and Care Digital Capabilities Framework. Health Education England, London.

Health Education England, 2019. The Topol Review: Preparing the Healthcare Workforce to Deliver the Digital Future. Health Education England, London. Available at: https://topol.hee.nhs.uk/.

Health Education England, 2021. Data Driven Healthcare in 2030: Transformation Requirements of the NHS Digital Technology and Health Informatics Workforce. Interim Report.

Nursing and Midwifery Council, 2018. Future Nurse: Standards of Proficiency for Registered Nurses. Available at: https://www.nmc.org.uk/globalassets/sitedocuments/standards-of-proficiency/nurses/future-nurse-proficiencies.pdf.

Nursing and Midwifery Council, 2019. Standards of Proficiency for Midwives. Available at: https://www.nmc.org.uk/globalassets/sitedocuments/standards/standards-of-proficiency-for-midwives.pdf.

OECD, 2016. Getting Skills Right: Assessing and Anticipating Changing Skill Needs. OECD Publishing, Paris. https://doi.org/10.1787/9789264252073-en.

Royal College of Nursing, 2018. Every Nurse an E-Nurse: Insights from a Consultation on the Digital Future of Nursing. RCN, London.

The Consultancy, 2021. Digital Literacy in the UK: Employer Perspectives and the Role of Higher Education. Times Higher Education, London.

UNESCO, 2011. Digital Literacy in Education. Policy Brief. Available at: http://unesdoc.unesco.org/images/0021/002144/214485e.pdf.

Wachter, R.M., 2016. Making IT Work: Harnessing the Power of Health Information Technology to Improve Care in England. Report of the National Advisory Group on Health Information Technology in England. William Lea Crown.

WHO, 2020. State of the World's Nursing 2020: Investing in Education, Jobs and Leadership. World Health Organisation, Geneva.

WHO, 2021. Global Strategic Directions for Nursing and Midwifery 2021–2025. World Health Organisation, Geneva.

CHAPTER 5

Specialist Roles and Competence

Natasha Phillips ■ Dionne Rogers ■ Sarah Hanbridge
■ Jen Bichel-Findlay

LEARNING OUTCOMES

At the end of this chapter, the nurses will be able to:

- Discuss the evolution and future potential of digital nurse practice.
- Develop a critical awareness of the ways nurses develop the knowledge and skills for these roles.
- Examine their digital health capabilities and learning needs through a relevant competency framework.

Introduction

This chapter provides an overview of the emergent field of specialist digital nursing practice. It then examines the ways nurses prepare for these roles, considering formal education and competency frameworks as tools for developing expertise in this speciality. Global variation is considered in the approaches to developing nurses with the expertise to lead in the development of digital healthcare solutions that support nursing practice and patient outcomes. Finally, organisations and networks that support nurses practising in and learning about this speciality are introduced. Learning exercises are used to support the reader in considering their own personal d evelopment as a digital nurse specialist. Globally, as the demand for and the cost of healthcare rises, the need to deliver the Triple Aim, developed by the Institute for Health Improvements, of improving the experience of care, improving population health and reducing costs of healthcare (Berwick et al. 2008), becomes more urgent. Recently, it has been proposed that this be expanded to a quintuple aim, incorporating workforce wellbeing and advancing health equity (Nundy et al. 2022). The use of digital technologies and data science has the potential to enable the healthcare systems to deliver all these aims. The rapid adoption of new technologies and data science is resulting in the need for a significant expansion of a specialist clinical workforce to ensure their implementation delivers the quintuple aim. Nurses are ideally placed to take up this specialist work, given their comprehensive understanding of the care environment.

While the whole nursing profession needs to be aware of, and skilled in, the use of technology and data in relation to health outcomes, additional knowledge and skills are needed by those tasked with leading the digital healthcare transformation. There are a variety of roles and titles for these expert nurses. However, in this chapter, we refer to them collectively as digital nurse specialists.

EVOLVING SPECIALIST NURSE ROLES – THE RISE OF THE NURSE INFORMATICIAN

Specialist roles for nurses leading the adoption of digital technologies to support care delivery initially appeared in the 1980s; the term nurse informatician was coined in 1992 in the United States (US) to describe this speciality. This specialty is in varying degrees of maturity globally, but the title nurse informatician has been picked up by other nations. Thus, currently, nurse informatician is the most widely understood description for nurses specialising in digital healthcare. There are a variety of definitions of nurse informatician, arguably in part due to the rapid pace of evolution of digital technologies in healthcare and the breadth of practice they cover. One of the most comprehensive definitions is captured in the American Nurses Association (ANA 2015: 1–2) Nursing Informatics: Scope and Standards of Practice.

> *Nursing Informatics is the speciality that integrates nursing science with multiple information and analytical sciences to identify, define, manage and communicate data, information, knowledge and wisdom in nursing practice. NI supports nurses, consumers, patients, the interprofessional healthcare team, and all other stakeholders in their decision-making in all roles and settings to achieve desired outcomes. This support is accomplished through the use of information structures, information processes, and information technology.*

This definition captures the uniqueness of nursing informatics, distinguishing it from other clinical informatics role by highlighting the importance of bringing nursing expertise, alongside expertise in technology and data science. It also goes some way to capturing the breadth of the speciality, pointing to the need to support the wider profession through the development and adoption of appropriate technologies and information structures to support care delivery across all settings. This breadth means that there is not only a multiplicity of roles for nurses seeking to practise this speciality, but also a variety of scope in how nurses individually span practice, research, education and leadership.

Working across the whole spectrum of nursing practice and care settings, the digital nurse specialist advises digital health teams on nursing workflow and requirements, develops resources and toolkits to support digital health implementations, contributes to the design of systems and interfaces, and ensures that systems and workflows adhere to digital health standards. Combining their nursing expertise with informatics expertise, they understand and communicate the reason behind new systems and processes that rely on technology; they also support the implementation of new processes and validate data quality from new technologies and processes (Hübner et al. 2022). This involves providing expertise in nursing documentation standardisation, process re-engineering, information management, and advocating for needs that will improve the experience of care delivery for nurses, such as devices that are integrated, voice and biometric activated, handheld, portable, wireless, capable of auto population and 'smart'. To this end, they assist in the development of nomenclatures, vocabularies, classifications, terminologies and minimum datasets that assist in the integration of information systems into the daily workflow of nursing care delivery (Hübner et al. 2022). All these endeavours support not only nurses in practice, but also impact the outcomes and experience of patients and the efficiency of care delivery.

The senior role of the Chief Nursing Informatics Officer (CNIO) emerged in the US as a strategic leadership role responsible for the safe implementation of technology in healthcare organisations and systems. Bridging the gap between information technology staff, clinicians and management, CNIOs lead critical initiatives that influence improved clinical efficiencies for all disciplines, not just nurses. They are strategic partners in the planning and implementation of new models of care that leverage technology, as well as in evaluating organisational infrastructure that supports these new models (Ventura 2018). The CNIO is well positioned to strengthen informatics and clinical analytics capacity across the healthcare workforce and to verify that nursing clinical information system and workflow requirements minimise the potential for adverse events and maximise the delivery of safe quality care (Australian College of Nursing 2022).

In addition to nursing, technical and data science expertise, the CNIO needs advanced leadership skills to work as part of a wider team to deliver the digital vision of a healthcare organisation. Primarily advocating for nurses, this leader needs to be skilled in successfully responding to societal, economic and political challenges that frequently occur in contemporary healthcare settings (Australian College of Nursing 2022). CNIOs are responsible for raising the profile of informatics within nursing practice, education and research and work with nurse leaders to champion the inclusion of digital technologies and data science across these domains. Leading nursing through technology transformation and interdisciplinary data analysis relies on innovative change and project management skills, aligned with the organisational vision, mission and strategic goals. Working together as strategic leaders, CNIOs have the potential to deliver system-wide changes, facilitating the development of a nursing career pathway with embedded digital health education in undergraduate and postgraduate courses of study and of onboarding and in-service programs, and ensuring continuous professional development of all nurses (Australian College of Nursing 2022).

While the title has been taken up globally, the role is enacted and operates at very different levels across different healthcare systems. In the UK, efforts are underway to standardise this as a strategic role for a senior nurse (National Health Service England 2022). Efforts have been made to standardise descriptions of these roles globally; notably, the Healthcare Information and Management Systems Society (HIMSS) standardised CNIO job description (HIMSS 2020). The standardisation of roles, job descriptions, competencies and education are considered vital to both the effective delivery of digital transformation and the development of a professional workforce that is able to do so. It is unsurprising then that the literature is full of articles outlining efforts to achieve this since the inception of nursing informatics in 1992. Nevertheless, it is disappointing that widespread variation continues to exist. Encouragingly, these efforts are gaining pace as digital healthcare accelerates; however, more needs to be achieved to ensure that specialist nursing workforce growth and preparation keeps pace with changes in healthcare enabled by technology.

PREPARING SPECIALIST DIGITAL NURSES FOR PRACTICE – FORMAL EDUCATION

There is wide variation in how nurses are prepared for specialist digital roles, and many nurses report falling into these roles by accident and learning on the job. Globally, defined roles and standards for practice vary, as does the education of nurses to work as digital specialists. In some countries, postgraduate qualifications in health informatics exist, but these are not a requirement for practice. In the US, however, certification as an informatics nurse is well established via the American Nurses Credentialing Center (ANCC). Nurses who evidence the practice requirements and successfully complete an examination are credentialled as 'Registered Nurse-Board Certified'. This approach is underpinned by formal education which has abounded in the US since the 1990's. These programmes are underpinned by 16 defined standards of practice (ANA 2015). These standards underpin the available education programmes and thus ensure a consistent standard of education and ultimately, practice, thereby leading to better outcomes for patients.

In contrast, specialist nursing informatics postgraduate programmes do not exist in the UK, though more generic programmes, like health informatics and digital healthcare master's degrees, are available (Health Education England (HEE) 2017). These programmes offer a breadth of knowledge pertaining to informatics and digital transformation in healthcare, but do not offer nursing knowledge alongside other knowledge domains. Instead, they rely on the learner to situate their learning in the context of their professional nursing practice.

Hanson and Hamric (2003) suggest that specialist practice emerges in response to a need in healthcare systems and evolves into advanced practice over time. They define these in three evolutionary stages: 1) Specialty develops in practice settings; 2) Organized training for specialty begins and 3) Knowledge base grows, which mounts pressures for standardization, subsequently leading to the emergence of graduate educational programs. Arguably, digital nurse specialist practice has emerged in response to the need for digital healthcare, but is at different stages of the advanced practice evolution globally, having reached stage 3 in the US. This evolution indicates that advanced practice should be considered as a framework for career pathways and when developing education for digital nurse specialists. Advanced clinical practice has been defined as practice that:

'is delivered by experienced, registered health and care practitioners. It is a level of practice characterised by a high degree of autonomy and complex decision making. This is underpinned by a masters level award or equivalent that encompasses the four pillars of clinical practice, leadership and management, education and research, with demonstration of core capabilities and area specific clinical competence'.

(HEE 2017: 8)

Advanced nursing practice is global and while there are variations, the International Council of Nurses Advanced Practice Network has reached a consensus on a definition suggesting that both expanded practice and expert knowledge shaped by practice are the core features of advanced practice. Like HEE, they also recommend that a master's degree be required for entry level of advanced practice.

In conclusion, approaches to formal education for digital nurse specialists vary globally. Adopting the pillars of advanced practice underpinned by existing competencies/standards of practice (discussed in next section) can ensure the standard of digital nurse education. This has both the potential to deliver a skilled specialist workforce needed and provide an attractive defined career pathway for nurses who choose this specialism. In the meantime, organisations and individuals should consider informal and work-based education to ensure competence when practising in this field.

Competencies

It is widely recognised that all healthcare professionals including nurses need competence to work in a digital healthcare system (Topol 2019; Wachter 2016). As far back as 2001, Staggers et al. sought to identify the competencies needed by nurses to work with digital technologies. Several frameworks have emerged that highlight the competencies required by all nurses. These also stratify levels of competence in an effort to indicate the additional competencies required by those working as specialists (Australian Digital Health Agency 2020; HEE 2017). Though early competencies defined by Staggers et al. (2001) have been evaluated to some extent, there has been limited evaluation of either the content or the impact of latest competency frameworks. This is an area for further research to enable specialist nurses, healthcare organisations and education providers to determine the best framework to underpin practice and education. This should also be considered alongside the ANA standards for practice which have underpinned nursing informatics education in the US since 1992.

Competency frameworks perform several key functions in relation to ensuring the advanced standard of practice of digital nurse specialists. They can be used to underpin the job descriptions, perform appraisals, inform personal development plans and design curricula for programmes of education that prepare students for the role. In addition, and in line with professional codes of conduct, it is vital that digital nurse specialists take responsibility for their own learning. Assessing themselves against available competency frameworks is a first step in identifying learning needs and opportunities to address these needs.

LEARNING EXERCISE

Pick a competency framework and map your own digital literacy with the domains therein. Where do you sit on the spectrum between novice and expert across the domains?

Now consider, as a digital nurse specialist, where you would place nursing colleagues in your own organisation on this spectrum. How as an 'expert' might you plan to upskill your colleagues?

A recent example of a competency framework entirely focused on the specialist practitioner is the UK Faculty of Clinical Informatics competency framework (Davies et al. 2022). This was developed in collaboration with many clinical informaticians and has again defined competencies needed by all clinicians, including nurses, specialising in this field (Davies et al. 2022). The framework is structured around six key areas: health and wellbeing in practice, information technologies and systems, working with data and analytical models, enabling human and organisational change, decision-making, leading informatics teams and projects. These competencies go beyond the technical, covering a complex array of clinical, technical, data, leadership and change management skills required of nurses and other clinicians seeking to practice this speciality. Another example targeted at nurses was developed by HIMSS Technology Informatics Guiding Education Reform (TIGER) committee.

Despite a plethora of competency frameworks, a recent systematic review recommended that a unified competency framework be developed to standardise the required knowledge and skills for the clinical informatics profession (Davies et al. 2021). This focus on defining and redefining competence does not appear to be leading to the widespread standardisation of roles and education programmes beyond the US. The World Health Organization (WHO) established a call for experts in early 2023 to contribute to the development of a digital health competency framework that will strengthen the capacity at the country level, as well as guide curriculum developers, leaders, policymakers, planners and practitioners (WHO 2023). Competency frameworks should be live documents reflecting changing practice and it is important that efforts to advance this relatively new nursing speciality focus on making these frameworks living, breathing tools that support nurses to grow and advance their practice.

LEARNING EXERCISE

Map your own knowledge and experience to the FCI competency framework. Identify strengths and gaps. Consider do you need the breadth of skills needed across the six domains and how would you build a personal development plan to address gaps?

Informal Education

As specialist nursing practice in digital transformation grows, so do the organisations and networks supporting these specialists to expand their expertise. Organisations like Healthcare Information and Management Systems Society (HIMSS), the College of Healthcare Information Management Executives (CHIME), and the Australasian Institute of Digital Health (AIDH) offer networks and learning, and have developed certification programmes to evidence expertise in this field. While these may lack the depth of more formal academic studies, they are supported by competencies. National nursing organisations, like the American Nursing Credentialing Centre (ANCC), Australian Nursing and Midwifery Federation (ANMF) and Royal College of Nursing (RCN), are articulating their position on the impact of digital healthcare on nursing and the role of nurses in digital healthcare. They are developing resources to support the general nursing workforce and those in specialist roles or those seeking to enter the field. In addition, specialist organisations like the American Medical Informatics Association (AMIA), European Federation for Medical Informatics (EFMI), AIDH, and International Medical Informatics Association (IMIA) seek to advance this field of specialist practice by generating evidence to inform practice and bringing communities together through mediums like academic conferences and journals to share this learning. All these organisations are instrumental in not only supporting current practice but also advocating for and advancing specialist nursing practice in digital healthcare for the benefit of the profession and the people it serves across all care settings. Nurses specialising in digital healthcare should explore and become involved in those organisations that best reflect their interests.

LEARNING EXERCISE

Using the resource list at the end of this chapter, explore the organisations and networks that support digital healthcare specialists. Consider how you might participate in one or some of these organisations to grow your expertise in this speciality.

CASE STUDY

Joy started a career in nursing over 20 years ago, when the use of technology in education or for care delivery was limited; digital literacy was not a feature of her pre or post registration training. As her career progressed and with increasing availability of technology, wide ranging digital roles and opportunities to engage in digital programmes emerged. Joy is now in a digital nurse specialist role, supporting the digital literacy development of other healthcare professionals. Her other interest is in artificial intelligence and how that can be used to develop screening tools to support maintenance of mental well-being. Joy is pursuing this interest through the NHS Clinical Entrepreneur programme. Her experiences have been enabled by supportive working environments and leaders. Formal recognition for the knowledge and skills acquired through these experiences cannot currently be captured by professional or regulatory processes.

Future Evolution/Conclusion

It is imperative that nurses have access to technology and information that can help them assess the recipients of care more accurately, resulting in improved decision-making and health outcomes. The ever-growing digitisation of healthcare requires nurses with knowledge and understanding of how to use technology and data to solve problems and positively impact care delivery for the recipients.

As technology advances rapidly, it is likely that new capabilities will be needed across nursing and wider clinical workforce. These are poorly understood but are likely to lead to changes in the way nurses practice, expanding roles to include digital health and information navigation that support people to use technologies, as well as to understand and use health information to be active partners in their care (Wisniewski et al. 2020).

Digital transformation requires some nurses to specialise in this field, developing expertise in digital technologies and data science for healthcare. These nurses must not only have specialist technical skills but also be prepared to advocate for practical technological processes that support busy nurse workloads, strengthen existing workflows, create aligned new workflows, and deliver effective care and health outcomes. To ensure the best possible outcomes of digital transformation for nurses and the people they serve, this specialist practice needs nurses to work as a global community to develop and grow the speciality and shape education that is underpinned by standards of competent practice.

Key Points

1. Nursing Informatics roles first emerged in the 1980s and are evolving in response to the rapid development of digital technologies and data science to support care delivery.
2. Specialist nurses with expertise in technology and data science are vital for ensuring that digital transformation delivers the benefits of the quintuple aim.
3. Approaches to education for this 'specialism' vary globally and many nurses entering this field rely on experiential learning to develop expertise.
4. There are a variety of competency frameworks to support those who wish to develop in this specialism. These are valuable for self-assessing and identifying learning needs and should underpin learning activities, including formal programmes of education.
5. There are a variety of education opportunities, formal and informal, available to support nurses who wish to pursue a career as a digital nurse specialist. To ensure safe practice, standards of education underpinned by the pillars of advanced practice should be adopted globally.

References

American Nurses Association (ANA), 2015. Nursing Informatics: Scope and Standards of Practice, second ed. Silver Spring, Maryland.

Australian College of Nursing (ACN), 2022. Leading Digital Health Transformation: The Value of Chief Nursing Information Officer (CNIO) Roles. Canberra: ACN. Available at: https://www.acn.edu.au/wp-content/uploads/position-statement-leading-digital-health-transformation-value-cnio-roles.pdf.

Australian Digital Health Agency (ADHA), 2020. National Nursing and Midwifery Digital Health Capability Framework. ADHA, Sydney. Available at: National_Nursing_and_Midwifery_Digital_Health_Capability_Framework_publication.pdf.

Berwick, D.M., Nolan, T.W., Whittington, J., 2008. The triple aim: care, health, and cost. Health Aff. 27 (3), 759–769. https://doi.org/10.1377/hlthaff.27.3.759.

Davies, A., Hassey, A., Williams, J., et al., 2022. Creation of a core competency framework for clinical informatics: from genesis to maintaining relevance. Int. J. Med. Inf. 168, e104905. https://doi.org/10.1016/j.ijmedinf.2022.104905.

Davies, A., Mueller, J., Hassey, A., et al., 2021. Development of a core competency framework for clinical informatics. BMJ Health & Care Informatics 28, e100356. https://doi.org/10.1136/bmjhci-2021-100356.

Hanson, C.M., Hamric, A.B., 2003. Reflections on the continuing evolution of advanced practice nursing. Nurs. Outlook 51 (5), 203–211. https://doi.org/10.1016/S0029-6554(03)00158-1.

Health Education England (HEE), 2017. Multi-professional Framework for Advanced Clinical Practice in England. Available at: https://www.hee.nhs.uk/sites/default/-files/documents/multi-professionalframeworkforadvancedclinicalpracticeinengland.pdf.

Healthcare Information and Management Systems Society (HIMSS), 2020. Chief Nursing Informatics Officer Job Description. Available at: https://www.himss.org/sites/hde/files/media/file/2020/12/08/himss-cnio-job-description-2020-final.pdf.

Hübner, U.H., Wilson, G.M., Morawski, T.S., et al., 2022. Nursing informatics through the lens of interprofessional and global health informatics. In: Hübner, U.H., Wilson, G.M., Morawski, T.S., Ball, M.J. (Eds.), Nursing Informatics: A Health Informatics, Interprofessional and Global Perspective, fifth ed. Springer, Cham.

National Health Service England (NHSE), 2022. Guidance for nursing on 'what good looks like'. Available at: https://transform.england.nhs.uk/digitise-connect-transform/what-good-looks-like/guidance-for-nursing-on-what-good-looks-like/.

Nundy, S., Cooper, L.A., Mate, K.S., 2022. The quintuple aim for health care improvement: a new imperative to advance health equity. JAMA 327 (6), 521–2. https://doi.org/10.1001/jama.2021.25181.

Staggers, N., Gassert, C.A., Curran, C., 2001. Informatics competencies for nurses at four levels of practice. J. Nurs. Educ. 40 (7), 303–316. https://doi.org/10.3928/0148-4834-20011001-05.

Topol, E., 2019. The topol review: preparing the healthcare workforce to deliver the digital future. Health Education England, London. Available at: https://topol.hee.nhs.uk/the-topol-review/#:~:text=The%20Topol%20Review%20outlined%20recommendations%20to%20ensure%20the,greater%20scale%20than%20anywhere%20else%20in%20the%20world.

Ventura, R., 2018. The Role of the Chief Nursing Informatics Officer: Position Statement of the American Nursing Informatics Association Board of Directors. Available at: https://www.ania.org/assets/documents/position/cnioPosition.pdf.

Wachter, R.M., 2016. Making IT Work: Harnessing the Power of Health Information Technology to Improve Care in England. Report of the National Advisory Group on Health Information Technology in England. Available at: https://assets.publishing.service.gov.u

k/government/uploads/system/uploads/attachment_data/file/550866/Wachter_Review_Accessible.pdf.

Wisniewski, H., Gorrindo, T., Rauseo-Ricupero, N., et al., 2020. The role of digital navigators in promoting clinical care and technology integration into practice. Digit. Biomark. 4 (Suppl. 1), 119–135. https://doi.org/10.1159/000510144.

World Health Organization (WHO), 2023. Open Call for Experts to Serve as Members of the Digital Health Competency Framework Committee. Available at: https://www.who.int/news-room/articles-detail/open-call-for-experts-to-serve-as-members-of-the-digital-health-competency-framework-committee.

Further Resources

American Nurses Credentialing Centre (ANCC). Nursing informatics certification. Available at: https://www.registerednursing.org/certification/nursing-informatics/.

American Medical Informatics Association (AMIA). About ANI. Available at: https://www.allianceni.org/about-us.

American Medical Informatics Association (AMIA). Nursing informatics. Available at: https://amia.org/communities/nursing-informatics.

Australasian Institute of Digital Health (AIDH). Nursing and midwifery digital health network. Available at: https://digitalhealth.org.au/nursing-and-midwifery/.

CHIME International. Education and accreditation. Available at: https://www.chimeinternational.org/home#education.

European Federation for Medical Informatics (EFMI). NI – nursing informatics. Available at: https://efmi.org/workinggroups/ni-nursing-informatics/.

Health Education England (HEE). Advanced practice. Available at: https://advanced-practice.hee.nhs.uk/.

Health Information and Management Systems Society (HIMSS). TIGER virtual learning environment. Available at: https://www.himss.org/tiger-virtual-learning-environment.

Faculty of Clinical Informatics. The faculty of clinical informatics. Available at: https://facultyofclinicalinformatics.org.uk/.

International Medical Informatics Association (IMIA). IMIA NI. Available at: https://imia-medinfo.org/wp/sig-ni-nursing-informatics/.

Royal College of Nursing. eHealth forum. Available at: https://www.rcn.org.uk/Get-Involved/Forums/eHealth-Forum.

CHAPTER 6

Leadership for Successful Digital Transformation

Natasha Phillips ▪ Louise Cave ▪ Helen Crowther ▪ Aaron Jones

LEARNING OUTCOMES

At the end of this chapter, the nurses will be able to:
- Discuss organisational and leadership theories and their application to their own practice.
- Consider the relationship between organisational context and individual leadership.
- Critically evaluate collective leadership as an approach to advancing nursing practice.
- Describe how collective leadership can enable successful digital transformation.

Introduction

Nurses, like other healthcare workers across the globe, are under significant stress and at risk of burnout (World Health Organization 2019). This has resulted in poor retention rates and regular reports of nurses having poor job satisfaction. Digital healthcare has been seen as one solution to addressing the challenges that have led to burnout and stress. However, to date, nurses have been poorly served by digital technologies; they report poor preparation for, and increased workload from using technologies, such that they perceive technology adds no value (Wisner et al. 2019). Despite this, digital transformation in healthcare is moving at a rapid pace, affecting nurses across all areas of practice and care settings. Leadership within the profession is required to effectively deliver the size and scale of change necessary for care delivery while meeting the needs of the nursing workforce. This leadership needs to come from all levels of the nursing workforce, including executive nurse leaders, digital specialist nurses and point of care nurses. This chapter examines how collective leadership approaches within and across organisations can be adopted to meet the challenges posed by digital transformation in healthcare.

This chapter introduces leadership and organisational theories. The principles of collective leadership are introduced, and different approaches are examined. The value of collective leadership in delivering large-scale organisational change is discussed and the benefit of this leadership approach for digital transformation specifically is considered. Case studies and learning exercises are embedded throughout, to enable nurses to see how they can embrace collective leadership to deliver change in their own settings.

Leadership in Context

Digital transformation, like all changes, occurs in the context of organisations. Dominant organisational theory conceptualises organisations as systems (Schein 1992). This theory is widely adopted in healthcare organisations and reflects dominant approaches to managing healthcare and associated change programmes. Here, the leader applies tools and techniques, like vision and strategy and policy and process to manage 'the system' (Burke 2018). An alternative radical social theory conceptualises organisations as complex responsive processes of relating (Stacey 2012). From this perspective, the work of organisations is achieved through the ongoing local interdependent human interaction of people working in them (Phillips 2020). From this perspective, the leader is part of the organisation where attention to both the quality of the conversation and those included in the conversation is important (see Table 6.1).

LEARNING EXERCISE

Consider your own experience of leading change in healthcare. What features of systems and complexity theory existed? How did they impact your ability to deliver the change?

In highly complex healthcare organisations, it is evident that leadership of digital transformation cannot be left to a few digital nurse specialists. Instead, it requires the collective leadership of many. Working as part of a digital multi-disciplinary team, the digital nurse specialist will need to mobilise the profession, from executive nurses to those at the point of care, ensuring they enact their leadership across all parts of the health and care system.

Leadership Styles

In this scenario, where large-scale change in the context of complex healthcare organisations and systems is under way, the individual leader should consider their own approach to leading. Leadership has long been an area of concern for the profession and several leadership styles have been advocated, including transformational (McGuire 2006), congruent (Stanley 2006), and, more recently, shared or distributed leadership (Turnbull-James 2011). This distributed approach is also referred to as collective leadership (West et al. 2014).

The limitation of the most widely advocated approach, transformational leadership, is the risk of digital nurse specialists adopting the mantle of leader as 'hero'.

TABLE 6.1 ■ **A Comparison of the Features of Two Theories of Organisations**

Systems Theory	Complexity Theory
Individuals are independent and autonomous.	Individuals are interdependent, not autonomous.
The organisation is a social system that exists outside the individual.	Individuals communicate through the conversation of gestures, not sender/receiver.
The system is a living thing that is affected by its environment.	These interactions constitute figurations of power.
Change in the system is caused by autonomous leaders.	Ideologies emerge in these processes of power relating.
Dual causality.	Ideologies constrain and enable conversation.
The system can be controlled and homeostasis can be achieved.	Ideologies sustain and change power relating patterns.
This control is achieved through the application of the tools and techniques of rational science.	The future is 'predictably unpredictable', emerging as global patterns from local interaction.
	Organisations are emergent, created in the interactions of interdependent individuals.
	No dual causality, but paradox – both at the same time.

Adapted from Phillips' (2017) Unpublished Thesis.

Ultimately, this leadership approach leads to the risk of decision fatigue and burnout (Turnbull-James 2011). Instead, the digital nurse leader will need elements of all leadership approaches: the ability to create a shared vision and followership from transformational leadership, the authenticity that stems from connection with nursing values of congruent leadership, and the ability to involve others and distribute decision-making, as advocated in shared leadership approaches.

LEARNING EXERCISE

Now consider the leadership style. Which leadership theory does it most align to? How did this help or hinder the change you were leading? What was the impact on you and others?

Collective leadership recognises that leadership is not situated in an individual and is congruent with a theory of organisations as complex responsive processes of relating (Stacey 2012), where change is achieved in the ongoing interdependent interactions of all actors (Phillips 2017). It is an approach to developing a culture where leadership is distributed across an organisation (DeBrun and McAuliffe 2020). Collective leadership recognises the expertise of all and the need to harness this for a shared purpose, where everyone takes responsibility for the success of their organisation, not just their own role or area (West et al. 2014). This contrasts with approaches to leadership that focus on the capability of an individual leader while ignoring the interdependency of the collective workforce in delivering shared goals. A focus on harnessing and developing collective leadership recognises the expertise, capability, motivation and power in the collective. In healthcare organisations characterised by complexity, a culture of collective leadership can be fostered to ensure the delivery of nursing excellence in digital healthcare.

Developing Collective Leadership in Organisational Context

To effectively establish collective leadership and deliver change, the organisational context needs to be considered. There are several organisational development models developed from systems thinking that can be adopted for this. One such example is the Burke Litwin Model of Organisational Performance and Development (Burke 2018). Figure 6.1 illustrates the factors that contribute to organisational performance and successful change. These need to be considered to set the conditions for successful collective leadership.

An example of using this organisational development approach is the Magnet Model© or its sister programme, Pathway to Excellence©, both of which support organisations in delivering a shared goal: nursing excellence. The Magnet Model© (American Nurses Association 2022) has five organisational components that support outstanding clinical care environments: transformational leadership, structural empowerment, exemplary professional practice, new knowledge, innovations and improvements and empirical outcomes. Structural empowerment in the Magnet Model© is achieved through shared governance, which has four key components: partnership – emphasis on teamwork among nurses, healthcare providers and their patients; ownership – each team member owns their contribution to healthcare decision-making; equity – equal focus on services, patients and staff because each is essential in providing safe and effective care; and finally, accountability – considered the core of shared governance, it is the willingness to take responsibility for decision-making (Porter O'Grady 2009). Evidence suggests high levels of nurse engagement with shared governance improve patient outcomes and staff satisfaction (Kutney-Lee et al. 2016). However, achieving true shared governance can be challenging and requires outstanding nurse leadership to effectively establish collective leadership (Medeiros 2018). Nurse leaders must develop a recognition of the interdependence of the collective and use leadership skills that support effective conversation that surfaces difference of opinion and supports decision-making. This requires transformational, authentic leaders with the confidence and capability to establish the shared vision and to cede power to deliver it.

LEARNING EXERCISE

How would you go about implementing shared decision-making councils in your organisation? Who would you involve and what challenges do you foresee for individual leaders and the collective?

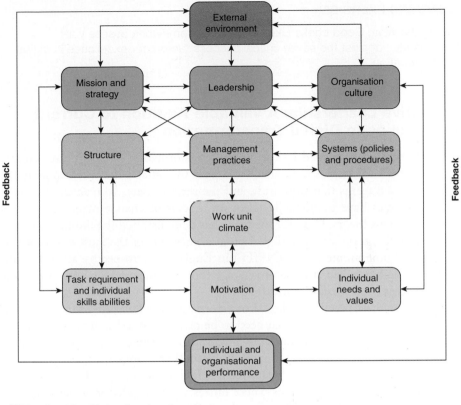

Fig. 6.1 **Burke Litwin model of organisational performance and development** (Adapted from Burke 2018).

Drawing on the evidence on organisational development, collective leadership and approaches like Magnet©, the Chief Nursing Information Officer (CNIO) for England implemented a strategy to create a culture of digital nursing excellence. Several collective leadership fora, including a national shared decision-making council of frontline digital nurse leaders, were established. The collective was used to define outstanding digital clinical practice environments and create an organisational framework for this; What Good Looks Like for Nursing (NHSE 2022) is an organisational development model that defines outstanding digital clinical practice environments where nursing excellence can flourish. The guidance incorporates 49 outcome-focused items serving as subscales for seven critical success factors: well-led, smart foundations, safe practice, supported people, empowered citizens, improved care and healthy populations. This model was launched for use in all organisations in England in 2022 and its impact is yet to be evaluated.

LEARNING EXERCISE

Using the What Good Looks Like for Nursing Framework, assess your organisation against the seven critical success factors for excellence in digital transformation.

Collective Leadership: A Valuable Addition to Current Approaches to Digital Transformation

The scale of change created by the digital transformation of healthcare requires large volumes of decisions to be made at a pace that affects the whole system, the individuals and teams that work in it, and the service users. To manage this scale, IT programmes have traditionally taken up models of change management that draw on systems theory. However, evidence has demonstrated the limitation of this approach with a series of failed digital programmes, one of the most famous being the national programme for IT (NPfIT) in England. Retrospective analysis demonstrated a failure called attention to engage those people working with systems to ensure success (Greenhalgh et al. 2011).

Since then, best practice in digital transformation includes involving end users in the multiplicity of decisions that need to be made to design and build technologies that meet their needs. Where this involvement occurs, programme outcomes like user adoption and staff experience are better. For example, a global report on user satisfaction with electronic health records (eHRs) found that there was higher nurse satisfaction in organisations where nurses were included in governance and decision-making (Jeppson 2022).

User centred design is central to digital programmes today and large-scale transformation of organisational structures and processes, often in the form of governance structures and design authority groups, are adopted to enable this. Case study one indicates how one healthcare system did this. While this shared decision-making has similarities with collective leadership, it fundamentally differs in that it uses the tools of systems thinking where power is in the leadership team convening the group. This contrasts with shared governance, where issues and ideas are encountered by frontline teams who are empowered to resolve them and escalate through shared governance councils to an executive leadership or programme board when local resolution is not possible.

Both shared decision-making through design authority groups and shared governance councils have their place in digital transformation. Case study one illustrates how design authority groups are established with a fixed end goal, while case study two illustrates how shared governance councils support an iterative approach of ongoing organisational conversations where practice issues are surfaced and addressed. To deliver ongoing sustainable digital transformation beyond the implementation of one system collective leadership across professions, organisations and systems must be culturally embedded. This requires digital nurse leaders with the insight, experience and expertise to lead in the context of healthcare systems characterised by complexity.

CASE STUDY: DESIGN WORKING GROUP

In New South Wales (NSW), Australia, the health system has a centralised pillar called eHealth NSW that is responsible for Information Communication and Technology and Digital Health. It supports 15 Local Health Districts (LHDs) and two Specialty Health Networks (SHNs) and a citizen population of 8.1 million. In recent times, the digitisation of the eHR in NSW has seen a State-based, standardised approach taken across all LHDs and SHNs to design eHR solutions. eHealth NSW established a governance model that brings together subject matter experts from across the state to ensure that design decisions are made by the best possible team of clinicians, consumers and other health staff. These groups are called Design Working Groups (DWGs) and they have the delegated authority to make clinical solution design decisions from the user perspective within a defined scope. The group works as a collective, with each member using their own unique background and experience to assist in the design and development of the eHR solution. The aim is to ensure that when the solution is implemented across NSW, it has had input from the right individuals to ensure that it is safe to use, patient centred and meets clinical requirements.

CASE STUDY: SHARED GOVERNANCE COUNCILS

A large NHS Trust in London moved from a multiplicity of systems for managing patient care to a single electronic health record, taking a big bang approach. Design authority working groups were established to manage the change. For nursing, the organisation had already adopted some principles of the Magnet Model to deliver nursing excellence. When faced with the challenge of moving all nurses from paper, a multiplicity of digital systems shared governance was harnessed and expanded to develop a nursing documentation shared governance council. All units and specialities were represented in this council who examined the current state of nursing documentation in the organisation and offered digital solution. Collectively, it was decided that the new system needed to support evidence-based nursing practice and represent the nursing process of assessing, planning, implementing and evaluating care to support excellence in patient care. The decision of this new council was taken to the executive nursing board, which approved the approach. However, this would require further investment and so, the nursing board endorsed and took this to the Trust executive board for approval and funding. Once approved, the responsibility to design the system was taken up by the nursing documentation council with its representation of local councils at ward/unit level. The council reported to executive nursing board, which dealt with issues the group could not resolve. This distribution of authority ensured that nurses identified the problems they wished to solve and were empowered to solve them as part of a large-scale organisational change. The documentation shared by the decision-making council was retained post implementation to maintain and iterate the digital documentation system in response to evolving practice and challenges that surfaced at the frontline.

Conclusion

This chapter outlined the importance of nurse leadership in digital transformation and introduced theories of leadership. The relationship between organisational structures and individual leadership was highlighted. The need for collective leadership was examined and shared governance was introduced as a structural tool to empower and engage nurses in digital transformation. Digital transformation must solve the real problems of nurses delivering care if it is to solve the complex challenges faced by healthcare systems and the populations they serve. This chapter argued that fostering a collective leadership culture creates an environment where empowered nurses can lead digital transformation. Furthermore, frameworks like Magnet Accreditation© and What Good Looks Like for Nursing (NHSE 2022) were introduced as structures and processes for creating outstanding digital clinical practice environments.

Key Points

1. Leadership of digital change in healthcare cannot be left to a few nurse specialists. Collective leadership is needed to deliver sustainable digital transformation of healthcare.
2. Healthcare systems are complex, nurses must use a breadth of leadership approaches to lead change in this context.
3. Organisational change models can help nurse leaders to understand this complexity and develop strategies for delivering change.
4. The What Good Looks Like Framework describes the core factors of successful digital transformation and is useful for delivering technology that supports the goals of healthcare.
5. Shared decision-making approaches are valuable for securing clinical engagement and shared ownership, collective leadership, of digital change.

References

American Nurses Association, 2022. Magnet Recognition Program | ANCC | ANA Enterprise. Available at: nursingworld.org.

Burke, W., 2018. Organizational Change: Theory and Practice, fifth ed. Sage Publications, Inc, Thousand Oaks, CA.

DeBrun, A., McAuliffe, E., 2020. Exploring the potential for collective leadership in a newly established hospital network. J. Health Organisat. Manag. 34 (4), 449–467. https://doi.org/10.1108/JHOM-12-2019-0353.

Greenhalgh, T., Russell, J., Ashcroft, R.E., et al., 2011. Why national eHealth programs need dead philosophers: wittgensteinian reflections on policymakers' reluctance to learn from history. Millbank Q. 89 (4), 533–563. https://doi.org/10.1111/j.1468-0009.2011.00642.x.

Jeppson, J., 2022. Arch Collaborative Nursing Guidebook 2022. Available at: https://klasresearch.com/archcollaborative/report/arch-collaborative-nursing-guidebook-2022/452.

Kutney-Lee, A., Germack, H., Hatfield, L., et al., 2016. Nurse engagement in shared governance and patient and nurse outcomes. J. Nurs. Adm. 46 (11), 605–612. https://doi.org/10.1097/NNA.0000000000000412.

McGuire, E., Kennerly, S.M., 2006. Nurse managers as transformational and transactional leaders. Nurs. Econ. 24 (4), 179–186.

Medeiros, M., 2018. Shared governance councils: 10 essential actions for nurse leaders. Nurs. Manag. 49 (7), 12–13. https://doi.org/10.1097/01.NUMA.0000538920.83653.9b.

National Health Service England (NHSE), 2022. Guidance for nursing on 'what good looks like'. Available at: https://transform.england.nhs.uk/digitise-connect-transform/what-good-looks-like/guidance-for-nursing-on-what-good-looks-like/.

Phillips, N., 2017. The Leadership Role of the NHS Ward Sister: A Case Study Informed by Complex Responsive Processes of Relating Unpublished Thesis. University of Hertfordshire, Hertfordshire.

Phillips, N., Norman, K., 2020. A case study of frontline nurse leadership informed by complex responsive processes of relating. J. Clin. Nurs. 29 (13–14), 2181–2195. https://doi.org/10.1111/jocn.15091.

Porter-O'Grady, T., 2009. Interdisciplinary Shared Governance: Structuring for 21st Century Practice Sudsbury. Jones & Bartlett, MA.

Schein, E.H., 1992. Organizational Culture and Leadership. Jossey Bass, San Francisco.

Stacey, R.D., 2012. Tools and Techniques of Leadership and Management: Meeting the Challenge of Complexity. Routledge, London.

Stanley, D., 2006. In command of care: toward the theory of congruent leadership. J. Res. Nurs. 11 (2), 132–144. https://doi.org/10.1177/1744987106059459.

Turnbull-James, K., 2011. The future of management and leadership in the NHS: no more heroes. In: Commission on Leadership & Management in the NHS. King's Fund, London. Available at https://www.kingsfund.org.uk/publications/future-leadership-and-management-nhs.

West, M., Eckert, R., Stewart, K., et al., 2014. Developing Collective Leadership for Health Care. King's Fund, London.

Wisner, K., Lyndon, A., Chesla, C.A., 2019. The electronic health record's impact on nurses' cognitive work: an integrative review. Int. J. Nurs. Stud. 94, 74–84. https://doi.org/10.1016/j.ijnurstu.2019.03.003.

World Health Organization, 2019. Burn-Out an 'Occupational Phenomenon': International Classification of Diseases. Available at: https://www.who.int/news/item/28-05-2019-burn-out-an-occupational-phenomenon-international-classification-of-diseases.

CHAPTER 7

Entrepreneurship in Nursing

Stacey Hatton ■ Emma Stanmore

LEARNING OUTCOMES

At the end of this chapter, the nurses will be able to:
- Understand the routes that nurses can take to drive innovation.
- Explain the value of nurses as entrepreneurs.
- Describe the barriers to entrepreneurship.
- Give examples of how healthcare organisations can promote entrepreneurship amongst nurses.

Introduction

Entrepreneurship within nursing, although evident in a variety of fields and settings, is a relatively unknown phenomenon, with scarce research on this subject.

The traditional perceptions of a nurse or midwife view them as female caregivers at the bedside of the patient. Commonly, the zero-error, risk-averse culture inherent in the nursing profession is seen as contradicting the pioneering, adaptable, risk-taking characteristics associated with entrepreneurs. Whilst these traditions might have appeared sufficient in the past, modern healthcare, with its increasing complexity and challenges, requires innovative solutions and ways of working to deliver more effective and efficient care.

One of the first and most prominent examples of a successful entrepreneurial nurse was Florence Nightingale, who revolutionised healthcare by utilising the power of science and data, and saved countless lives (Boore and Porter 2011). Since then, nurses have played a pivotal role in the area of innovation, digital health, data science and technologies, ensuring that solutions are fit for the purpose for patients, clinicians and organisations.

The relatively new digital nursing roles have been instrumental in influencing, changing and pioneering the digital advancements seen in healthcare today. The digital revolution is professed to be one of the most significant events in human history. The role of this chapter is to empower more nurses to lead in developing and adopting new digital technologies to advance patient-centred care and foster a culture of innovation and entrepreneurship.

How Can Nurses Innovate?

INTRODUCTION

Innovation is the process of change brought about by introducing new ideas, ways of working or products and services. Nurses around the world are frequently involved in innovative initiatives to improve patient care, outcomes and staff efficiencies. This section covers how nurses can innovate in the digital space by:

Cooperating with industry, suppliers and academics

Utilising internal IT resources

Developing solutions as an entrepreneur

Cooperating With Industry, Suppliers and Academics

Clinicians often endeavour to make changes in current processes or systems to positively influence patient outcomes and/or clinicians' workflows. Some organisations have adequate digital systems in place, whilst others require collaborative working with industry and academic partners and nurses in prime positions to lead changes in practice. For instance, the Digital Nurse roles support the digital transformation strategy in England. These specialists, alongside other innovators, utilise accredited suppliers and support the implementation of evidence-based digital tools to give providers more confidence in their route to digitisation.

Utilising Internal IT Resources

Nurses may also collaborate within their organisation and use internal resources to develop an 'in-house' solution. Defined by some as 'intrapreneurship', this activity takes place when an employee uses their creativity to develop services or products to make improvements in the organisation they work in, turning ideas into deliverable innovations (Neergard 2020). In the UK health system, the majority of entrepreneurial staff may take this route, particularly when supported by management. This route allows nurses to innovate without taking on financial or other risks.

Developing Solutions as an Entrepreneur

The most complex, but arguably the most rewarding way to innovate is to develop solutions as an entrepreneur.

An entrepreneur is defined as someone 'who organises, manages, and assumes the risks of a business or enterprise', with an enterprise being described, among others, as 'a project or undertaking that is especially difficult, complicated, or risky' (Neergard 2020). Within healthcare, the term social entrepreneurship is also used to describe entrepreneurial skills that are used to create and sustain not only commercial but also social values (Boore and Porter 2011). Therefore, entrepreneurship may encompass the development and translation of new innovations into practice as well as the commercialisation of a new product.

Entering the realm of developing new innovations and business ventures can be challenging for nurses as it requires preparation, knowledge, significant resources and experience outside of typical professional roles and education.

The odds of successfully navigating the journey from identifying an important unmet need to adopting an innovation as standard care can be increased if several steps

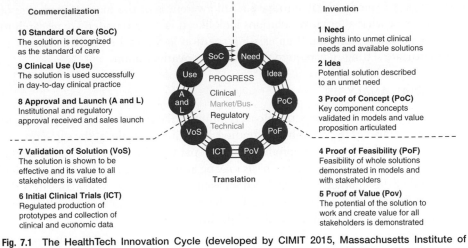

Commercialization

10 Standard of Care (SoC)
The solution is recognized
as the standard of care

9 Clinical Use (Use)
The solution is used successfully
in day-to-day clinical practice

8 Approval and Launch (A and L)
Institutional and regulatory
approval received and sales launch

7 Validation of Solution (VoS)
The solution is shown to be
effective and its value to all
stakeholders is validated

6 Initial Clinical Trials (ICT)
Regulated production of
prototypes and collection of
clinical and economic data

Invention

1 Need
Insights into unmet clinical
needs and available solutions

2 Idea
Potential solution described
to an unmet need

3 Proof of Concept (PoC)
Key component concepts
validated in models and value
proposition articulated

4 Proof of Feasibility (PoF)
Feasibility of whole solutions
demonstrated in models and
with stakeholders

5 Proof of Value (Pov)
The potential of the solution to
work and create value for all
stakeholders is demonstrated

Translation

Fig. 7.1   The HealthTech Innovation Cycle (developed by CIMIT 2015, Massachusetts Institute of Technology, Boston).

are taken before investing substantial amounts of time, money and other resources. The world leading Massachusetts Institute of Technology created a roadmap, known as the HealthTech Innovation Cycle (CIMIT 2015) to assist entrepreneurs in developing well-defined milestones/deliverables across clinical, market/business, regulatory and technical domains. Figure 7.1 gives an overview of these steps and further reading is recommended in the references section at the end of this chapter.

LEARNING EXERCISE

1. Consider an idea to improve an area of practice
2. Referring to the HealthTech Innovation Cycle (Fig. 7.1), how would you take this idea from concept to step 4 Proof of Feasibility?
3. What would you list as your top barriers or facilitators to progress your idea?

The areas listed below form a backbone of a basic plan, which can help with formulating the essential information required for the innovation and company. See the further readings in the references section for further information on these steps (Ries 2011).

INNOVATION OR BUSINESS JUSTIFICATION

Establishing an unmet need, a niche in the market or a problem that needs solving is usually the starting point for an individual to engage in the development of an innovation or business opportunity. There also needs to be a desire to implement the solution on a large scale rather than locally.

MARKET ASSESSMENT

Exploring the market is essential to gaining an appreciation of what solutions are already available, what is similar to your idea and how they differ. Although at this early stage it is rarely possible to have a full awareness of the market need, size of the market or what alternative solutions look like, it is vital to undertake research to gain even a limited picture. If an existing solution is found, its implementation in the healthcare setting may require significant innovative action.

FINANCIAL ANALYSIS

From a financial point of view, the most common initial route for a nurse midwife to commence a business is through self-funding. Working clinically at the same time as setting up and developing the product and company is challenging. Governmental innovation grants on a competitive basis may be available (see the references section at the end of this chapter). It is vital that an aspiring nurse thoroughly considers the time and finances that will be required for the product development and the enterprise to successfully function, sustain and grow.

TEAM

Understanding who is needed in your team in the early days is key. This might appear very simple, but few people truly appreciate the complexities that come with developing a new product or a start-up.

Involving users and stakeholders in the development of the solution and choosing resilient, consistent, positive, hard-working people is crucial for success. The size of the initial team may vary; however, in the case of digital innovations, a nurse may need the technical skills of a software engineer. This could potentially be achieved by presenting the engineers with the clinical problem and explaining how the innovation would solve it, as well as highlighting the value the cooperation could bring to them and to others. There are software engineers who are keen on cooperating with start-ups, and shares may be offered in return for their time and expertise.

IMPLEMENTATION TIMELINE

It is important to discuss with the engineer the time period to complete your first minimum viable product (MVP) and the length of time needed for a pilot and to implement your solution across a full department or organisation (depending on your product and goal).

FURTHER CONSIDERATIONS

It is paramount that before commencing an enterprise, an aspiring nurse acquires further knowledge and support in information governance, clinical safety standards, legal matters, including intellectual property rights, marketing, sales, funding and leadership.

This section covered the various ways in which a nurse can innovate. The next section explores the value the nurses represent, in the context of entrepreneurship.

The Value of Nurses as Entrepreneurs

While the transition from a nurse to an entrepreneur seems to involve contradictory values, cultures, working styles, and behaviours, both professions possess a diverse skillset that can be effectively transferred to health technology development business (Sharp et al. 2014; Vannucci et al. 2017; Wilson et al. 2012).

Nurses' attention to detail; ability to listen, manage their time effectively and prioritise their workload; as well as persistence and resilience, make them well suited for the challenges of developing a new technology and/or business venture.

In addition to their motivation and dedication to improving patient care, nurses are renowned for being empathetic team players. This feature is an invaluable asset, since modern businesses, especially IT, require seamless teamwork.

Nurses also possess a deep understanding of the clinical processes and have the clinical experience to direct the development of a solution; therefore, they are best placed to be at the heart of the innovation.

The three intrinsic human motivators – autonomy, mastery and purpose (Pink 2018) – are closely correlated with entrepreneurship. Many entrepreneurs set out on their journey in business because of a desire to serve a higher purpose and strive for something that has a greater impact.

Nurses' core values of care, dedication to patient care and commitment to the wellbeing of their colleagues amplify their commitment to the 'higher purpose', which makes them stand out as entrepreneurs.

Barriers to Entrepreneurship in Nursing

While nursing entrepreneurship dates back to Florence Nightingale, it is a rarely recognised phenomenon within the profession. This is surprising, considering the magnitude of the health IT industry and the unique value that nurses could bring to businesses.

There are layers of innovative potential within most clinical professionals; yet, stereotypical views of nurses and challenges present in the healthcare systems lead to barriers which prevent these professionals from pursuing entrepreneurial ventures.

LACK OF BUSINESS OR INNOVATION EXPERIENCE

One of the most obvious reasons that nurses avoid entrepreneurship is their lack of prior general business experience and relevant knowledge (Sharp et al. 2014). The complexity of legal matters and regulatory requirements (Elango et al. 2007) within the healthcare industry adds another layer of information that needs to be acquired, on top of general business skills.

LACK OF RESOURCES

Most nurses are in short supply of resources, such as time, money and others, necessary to pursue an entrepreneurial journey.

LACK OF ORGANISATIONAL SUPPORT

The healthcare sector has been described as being slow to adapt to the expanded nursing role. There is negligible training and number of structures at the level of hospitals, and very few on a national level, whose function is to support nursing entrepreneurship.

OUTDATED STEREOTYPES

Outdated stereotypes are another reason nurses do not to follow the path of entrepreneurship. Common perceptions of entrepreneurship lead some individuals to believe that combining business with the healthcare profession is contrary to nursing's caring values. Many clinical entrepreneurs encounter scepticism and are criticised for merging business with care (Neergard 2020). This leaves some nurses feeling less valued for pursuing entrepreneurial endeavours. Entrepreneurship is not the traditional nursing career path and as such, has been viewed as 'rebellious' or disloyal (Jakobsen et al. 2021).

TECHNOLOGY COMPETENCES

Working in today's multigenerational nursing profession means there is a difference in technology competencies between younger and older generation professionals (Rollan et al. 2021). Nurses who occupy decision-making positions may not understand the value that innovation in digital systems can bring to the patients, staff and an organisation as a whole. This could discourage an innovative nurse from showcasing their efforts to their peers and superiors.

This section explored many of the barriers that nurses face regarding entrepreneurship. The next section explores how these barriers can be overcome.

Organisations as Innovation Boosting Environment

INTRODUCTION

There are remarkable barriers to entrepreneurship amongst nurses. However, research suggests that these challenges can be overcome with '*coordinated action by individual nurses, professional associations, and public policy initiatives*' (Elango et al. 2007).

This section explores how healthcare and education organisations could break down those barriers and successfully foster entrepreneurship. In the presented framework, any nurse or midwife, at any point in their career, can receive substantial and meaningful support in inventing, prototyping, testing, implementing and scaling up a digital innovation. The main features of the proposed system are the low total cost of implementation, high result orientation, pragmatic approach and the emphasis on standardisation. If implemented methodically and with sufficient dynamism, such a framework could potentially bring enormous gains to the healthcare systems.

In addition to describing the components of the framework, the subsections below portray a chronologically ordered journey of a nurse entrepreneur.

There are several prerequisites for the programme to work:

- Nurses need to be **informed** about entrepreneurship being a valid and exciting option in their career, with enormous potential to benefit patients, at scale.
- Nurses must receive a theoretical **background knowledge** regarding innovation and entrepreneurship.
- Nurses must receive extensive **real-life exposure and practical support**.
- There must be a clear **incentivisation** scheme for all key people involved in promoting entrepreneurship and innovation.

Besides the points listed above, to ensure good cohesion, coordination and drive for the framework, there needs to be a person responsible for its implementation nationally.

LEARNING EXERCISE

Imagine you are a Chief Nurse or Chief Nursing Information Officer:
1. Consider how you might influence the development of new innovations in your organisation.
2. How would you ensure that you involve the perspectives of the frontline healthcare professionals?
3. How would you gain managerial buy-in?
Refer to the first Case Study for further guidance.

INFORMATION CAMPAIGN (3i)

For nurses to engage in entrepreneurship, there needs to be a well-organised campaign of informing, influencing, and incentivising (3i).

What to Communicate

Nurses need to know that the possibility of becoming an entrepreneur exists and is attractive.

They need to understand that the specific skills they possess make them best placed to pursue the entrepreneurial avenue, as discussed in the previous section.

Most nurses join the profession because they want to make a difference (Messineo et al. 2019). As entrepreneurs, they have an opportunity to make a difference on a bigger scale and have a greater impact on patient care and the wellbeing of nursing/midwifery staff.

The innovations of entrepreneurs could be valuable for the whole society and result in spectacular personal success for the nurse or midwife.

Who Could Communicate

Communication regarding entrepreneurship in nursing needs to be widespread across varying organisations. Starting from the top, those with authority in health-focused central governing bodies, hospitals, as well as academics of nursing/midwifery at universities would be essential.

This would be a huge stride forward in terms of breaking down the cultural barriers to nurse entrepreneurship.

Another group, crucial for the success of the framework, is the staff involved in innovation hubs, described further. These key people could deliver important messages to nurses to promote entrepreneurship and encourage their input in innovation projects.

Communication Channels

To effectively target potential nurse candidates, multiple communication channels could be utilised, including social media, journals and nursing/digital conferences.

It could also be potentially beneficial to incorporate a 1-day mini-course in the nursing university undergraduate programmes, as well as offer the optional 'Entrepreneurship in Nursing' course described further in the chapter.

To raise the profile of nursing entrepreneurship, the cyclical yearly/mandatory training could be enriched by a 15-minute session on entrepreneurship in nursing, led by the Innovation Hub staff, describing the options, the journey and the support available.

Theoretical Background Knowledge

The lack of business knowledge is a well-established and significant barrier to nurses pursuing entrepreneurial endeavours. To truly encourage these professionals to consider the prospect of turning an idea into business and then into value for patients and staff, help in this area must be very easy to access.

The two main components of the framework responsible for the delivery of the knowledge could be the Nursing Innovation Hubs and the 'Entrepreneurship in Nursing' course.

NURSING INNOVATION HUBS – THE INITIAL ROLE

Healthcare organisations can act in various ways to foster innovation and encourage nurses who wish to pursue entrepreneurship. A central point within each organisation could be a Nursing Innovation Hub (NIH). This would act as a doorway into the organisation for new nurse/midwife-led enterprises and allow innovative companies to enter the healthcare market.

To recruit talented innovators, NIHs should exist in every large healthcare organisation. Since the resources in healthcare are often scarce, the NMIH team could initially consist of just one dynamic, creatively thinking nurse working one day a week. This could be a person from the digital team or someone with a strong link with the Chief Nursing Informatics Office (CNIO), Chief Clinical Informatics Officer (CCIO) or the clinical digital team.

The initial role of the NIH would be purely informative, and the advice would be focused on providing the initial knowledge about the options for making an idea a reality, described in the 'How can nurses innovate' section. If the entrepreneurial route is considered, then a nurse would be given general basic business advice and information regarding the further steps.

ENTREPRENEURSHIP IN NURSING COURSE AND CERTIFICATION

After receiving initial information, a nurse/midwife could attend the Entrepreneurship in Nursing course. This course would provide them with essential general and health IT-specific knowledge and deliver pragmatic, step-by-step, standardised advice.

Such courses should be nationally supported and standardised with a curricula underpinned by defined competencies (see chapter 5).

To ensure high talent pickup, it is essential that the eligibility threshold be relatively low, with the course being accessible to every nursing professional. However, to allocate further resources to the best candidates, the course should be finalised with an exam and certification.

The subjects covered by the course could include legal matters, taxes, corporate governance, cyber security, information governance, HR, marketing, sales, funding, product development and clinical safety.

Real Life Exposure and Practical Support

There is nothing more difficult for an aspiring entrepreneur than finding a place to practically test and improve their innovation. This crucial role would be taken up by the NIH and each of the stages described below would be actively supported by the NIH staff.

INNOVATION HUBS – THE MAIN ROLE

After acquiring basic business knowledge, the next step for an entrepreneur is to discuss a proof of concept with a software engineer and create a prototype. There are multiple free and easy-to-use tools which can be used for this purpose and the NIH staff would advise on these (see the references section at end of chapter). This stage would also involve the entrepreneur creating an initial description of the value that the software would bring. After the prototype and the value proposition (reasons why the product/innovation would be used by service providers/patients/healthcare professionals) have been created, the clinical staff would need to be involved to refine both.

The next major phase in product development is creating a minimum viable product (for further reading, see Ries [2011] in the references section). This phase leads to a product that has a minimum number of features but is an end-to-end working software that can be tested to evaluate the technical reliability and gather feedback from the users. The basic rule at this stage is to involve a limited number of users and deploy the software in only one or two areas.

After refinements and thorough testing, the software may be ready to be deployed across the organisation. This stage gives an opportunity to gather more data from the users and carry out an economic evaluation to understand what significant benefits or return on investment the product can produce.

The successful organisation-wide deployment could lead to the scaling-up stage, where the solution is adopted by other organisations. This adoption could be facilitated by the NIH by informing other NIHs about its value.

Clinical Support

One of the key aspects of developing an innovation is collaboration and strong support from senior nursing staff, CNIO, other clinicians and academics (who can assist with rigorous evaluations and grant funding). To create a product which represents real value, clinicians need to engage by providing continuous feedback. The drive for this engagement should come from the highest levels of nursing management, who can also influence the strategic direction for product development.

Incentivisation Schemes

To ensure the effective functioning and success of the framework, targeted incentivisation schemes should be set up. The key people, essential for its success who should participate and benefit from the schemes, are the national coordinator, CNIOs, Directors and Deputy Directors of Nursing and the NIH staff.

On their part, the entrepreneurs should also incentivise the organisations by initially providing free or low-cost software, as well as, if possible, expertise and improvements to the hospital systems related to the software.

CASE STUDY

About

This case study relates to the company I co-founded and describes the journey we experienced from its inception to the first software deployment.

Background

I am currently a CNIO in the NHS in the UK, as well as in the company. Following many years of working in healthcare, a software engineer, a doctor and I joined forces to create a health IT enterprise developing quality assurance and improvement systems for healthcare.

Our First Client

When we approached the first acute hospital, now our exemplar site, we had a working but untested MVP and no real-life commercial IT experience.

We attended a meeting with the key stakeholders in the organisation and after seeing the product demo, the Deputy Chief Nurse, Sarah Ward, together with the Chief Digital Officer (CDO) and IT Director, made the decision to arrange a pilot.

The pilot was carried out in two surgical wards. We had regular progress meetings and, following user requests, made the necessary software improvements. After the pilot, the software went live in the surgical division and then across the whole organisation.

A realisation that cooperation with the company may bring multiple and scalable benefits to patient care prompted Sarah to establish regular meetings with us.

During the meetings, we received feedback from nurses on all managerial levels, which is crucial for developing innovative functionalities. Sarah has also, by providing us with valuable information about the hospital processes, effectively helped shape the strategic direction the company has taken. The regularity of the meetings gave us reassurance and a sense of stability so desired by inherently volatile start-ups.

The collaboration with our exemplar site continues to strengthen as we meet regularly to continue to improve our systems. We received overwhelmingly positive feedback and collaboratively carried out an economic evaluation, describing multiple areas in which the software improved patient care and staff efficiency.

During one of the recent meetings, the CDO of the hospital described our partnership as a blueprint for collaboration between a healthcare organisation and a start-up.

CASE STUDY: DEVELOPMENT OF A DIGITAL HEALTH APPLICATION INFORMED BY THE HEALTHTECH INNOVATION CYCLE (CIMIT 2015)

Need

Falls are a leading cause of emergency hospital admissions for older adults and are an increasing public health priority around the world. There is strong evidence that specific strength and exercise programmes can reduce falls by approximately a third. However, traditional exercise programmes can be costly, laborious, inaccessible to older adults, and limited by shortages of qualified professionals to deliver the training.

Idea for solution

A nurse-led academic collaboration with a tech-for-good company and with health and social care professionals was formed to develop a gamified tablet-based falls prevention application (KOKU app: https://kokuhealth.com). Successive grant funding was gained from a variety of research and development funders (ESRC, NHS England, Innovate UK) and University of Manchester support was obtained to complete development, perform research evaluations and create a business plan.

Proof of Concept

Users (older adults) and stakeholders (health and social care practitioners) were involved in the iterative development and testing until high usability and acceptability scores were obtained.

Proof of Feasibility

Real world testing in the community comprised a 6-week feasibility study that included baseline and 6-week questionnaires, qualitative focus groups and interviews.

Proof of Value

Regulatory approvals (clinical safety and GDPR General data Protection Regulations (EU legislation)) were obtained with the support of NHS Digital and a Community-Interest-Company was set up to sustain uptake and translation into practice.

Validation

Feasibility, usability and acceptability studies, and an implementation evaluation study were conducted with care providers in the Northwest of England. The evaluations demonstrated that KOKU is safe to use by older adults in their own home with trends in improvements seen after 12 weeks of use (3x per week) in multiple outcomes (e.g. reduced level of frailty and higher Quality of Life). This was further validated with qualitative feedback and independent studies by external organisations.

Post-study implementation of KOKU for older adults has continued and KOKU is now being scaled up and further evaluated as a digital health technology with large numbers of users.

Conclusion

There is a global nursing shortage, and healthcare systems are under substantial strain. This situation, however, coincides with a time of great technological advancements leading to increased staff efficiency, automated tasks, improved processes, thereby decreasing the amount of strain experienced by the healthcare systems. As an article on Forbes (Power 2021) noted, 'Entrepreneurs who bring disruptive innovations and ideas to the table, particularly when it comes to technology, can help the industry recover'.

To deliver these advancements, the industry needs digital solutions that are fit for purpose, future-proof, and are created with the involvement of users and frontline professionals.

If supported well, nurses can play a crucial role in developing these solutions. This, however, is only likely to happen if the nursing staff has easy access to well-organised support within a comprehensive framework organised by governing bodies and managers in the health sector. There is no better time than now for nurse innovators to step forward to accelerate developing and sustaining a culture of innovation and entrepreneurship.

LEARNING EXERCISE

Think about the biggest challenge you have in your work. Make notes on your answers to the following questions:
1. How would you approach this challenge as an innovator/entrepreneur?
2. Who might you need to work with to develop a possible solution?
3. What resources do you already have in-house and where might you go to obtain funding or further support or training?
4. How would you like your organisation to support you?

Key Points

1. The role of the nurse entrepreneur challenges the stereotypical view of the profession and has high value in meeting the demands of the challenges and complexities that the future of healthcare brings.
2. Nurses can innovate in several ways, including utilising internal IT resources, cooperating with industry, suppliers and academics to develop solutions as entrepreneurs.
3. Witnessing first-hand the problems in healthcare, frontline nurses possess unique values that are crucial for the development of innovative solutions. The diverse skillset that nurses hold makes them perfectly placed to pursue entrepreneurship.
4. Whilst there are significant barriers to entrepreneurship, these can be broken down when peers and organisations support individuals who choose this path.
5. Education, healthcare and government organisations can act in a variety of ways to promote and foster entrepreneurship amongst nurses. The effective framework for achieving this goal would likely consist of an information campaign, delivering theoretical knowledge to aspiring entrepreneurs, providing them with practical support and creating an incentivisation scheme for all key decision-makers.

References

Boore, J., Porter, S., 2011. Education for entrepreneurship in nursing. Nurse Educ. Today 31 (2), 184–191. https://doi.org/10.1016/j.nedt.2010.05.016.

Elango, B., Hunter, G., Winchell, M., 2007. Barriers to nurse entrepreneurship: a study of the process model of entrepreneurship. J. Am. Acad. Nurse Pract. 19 (4), 198–204. https://doi.org/10.1111/j.1745-7599.2007.00215.x.

Jakobsen, L., Qvistgaard, L., Trettin, B., et al., 2021. Entrepreneurship and nurse entrepreneurs lead the way to the development of nurses' role and professional identity in clinical practice: a qualitative study. J. Adv. Nurs. 77 (10), 4142–4155. https://doi.org/10.1111/jan.14950.

Messineo, L., Allegra, M., Seta, L., 2019. Self-reported motivation for choosing nursing studies: a self-determination theory perspective. BMC Med. Educ. 19 (1), 192. https://doi.org/10.1186/s12909-019-1568-0.

Neergard, G.B., 2020. Entrepreneurial nurses in the literature: a systematic literature review. J. Nurs. Manag. 29 (5), 905–915. https://doi.org/10.1111/jonm.13210.

Pink, D., 2018. Drive: The Surprising Truth About What Motivates Us. Riverhead Books, New York, NY.

Power, R., 2021. Healthcare Needs Entrepreneurs: Here Are 4 Ways to Future-Proof Your Innovations. Forbes. Available at: https://www.forbes.com/sites/rhettpower/-2021/09/26/healthcare-needs-entrepreneurs-here-are-4-ways-to-future-proof-your-innovations/?sh=66bc0ff1868f.

Rollan, S., Siles, J., 2021. Nursing professionals within the intergenerational context during the 20th and 21st centuries: an integrative review. Invest. Educ. Enfermería 39 (3), e14. https://doi.org/10.17533/udea.iee.v39n3e14.

Sharp, D.B., Monsivais, D., 2014. Decreasing barriers for nurse practitioner social entrepreneurship. J Am Assoc Nurse Pract. 26 (10), 562–566. https://doi.org/10.1002/2327-6924.12126.

Vannucci, M., Weinstein, S., 2017. The nurse entrepreneur: empowerment needs, challenges, and self-care practices. Nurs. Res. Rev. 2017 (7), 57–66. https://doi.org/10.2147/NRR.S98407.

Wilson, A., Whitaker, N., Whitford, D., 2012. Rising to the challenge of health care reform with entrepreneurial and intrapreneurial nursing initiatives. Online J. Issues Nurs. 17 (2), 1–12.

Further essential reading for start-up business support

Osterwalder, A., Pigneur, Y., 2010. Business Model Generation: A Handbook for Visionaries, Game Changers, and Challengers. John Wiley & Sons, Hoboken, New Jersey.

Ries, E., 2011. The Lean Startup. Crown Business, New York.

Company set up website information:

Gov.UK. Community interest companies: guidance chapters. Available at: https://www.gov.uk/government/publications/community-interest-companies-how-to-form-a-cic.

Gov.UK. Set up a limited company: step by step. Available at: https://www.gov.uk/set-up-limited-company.

Gov.UK. Setting up a social enterprise. Available at: https://www.gov.uk/set-up-a-social-enterprise.

Innovation grant funding websites:

For EU, see https://commission.europa.eu/research-and-innovation_en.

For UK, see https://www.ukri.org/councils/innovate-uk/ and https://sbrihealthcare.co.uk.

For USA, see https://www.nih.gov/grants-funding US grant database or https://www.grants.gov/web/grants/home.html.

Training:

For NHS Clinical Entrepreneur programme, see https://nhscep.com.

SECTION 3

Digitally Enabled Nursing and Midwifery Practice

CHAPTER 8

The Electronic Health Record: Opportunities and Challenges

Dawn Dowding ■ Loretto Grogan ■ Sarah Newcombe

LEARNING OUTCOMES

At the end of this chapter, the nurses will be able to:

- Understand nurses' role in the development, design and implementation of an Electronic Health Record.
- Have critical awareness of the organisational, human and technological factors that enable successful implementation of an Electronic Health Record.
- Evaluate the opportunities and challenges of implementing an Electronic Health Record.

Introduction

An Electronic Health Record (EHR) is a specific type of digital system that provides a longitudinal record of information about a person's health. Nurses spend the most time in direct patient care and collect a large volume of patient data, entering assessments, care plans and care notes into systems such as EHRs. High quality and thorough documentation of patient care are critical for patient safety, ensuring continuity of care via communication with other healthcare professionals and supporting nurses in reflecting and critically thinking about their patients' condition and responding to interventions. Clear, accurate, objective and timely record keeping is a fundamental part of the nursing code of practice.

Development and implementation of EHRs and other information technology offers significant opportunity to enhance nursing practice and the ability to evaluate and generate knowledge from nursing documentation. In this chapter, we discuss the factors that influence the successful implementation of an EHR and highlight the opportunities and challenges of using EHRs in a healthcare organisation. Although healthcare contexts and the types of EHR system implemented by healthcare organisations vary, there is a high degree of commonality across the critical factors for success derived from learning of successful and unsuccessful EHR implementations internationally. We highlight the key issues to consider, ensuring that EHR adoption supports nursing practice.

FACTORS FOR SUCCESSFUL EHR IMPLEMENTATION AND ADOPTION

An EHR is a complex type of digital technology introduced into a complex health-care environment. For it to be successful, a number of issues need to be considered, including:

- *organisational* factors, such as the role of leadership, training, resources and workflows;
- *human factors,* such as the skills of the workforce and interactions with the system and
- *technological factors,* such as how usable a system is, how well it communicates with other systems (interoperability) and infrastructure.

Organisational Factors

When thinking of introducing an EHR system, it must be noted that it is more than just a process of software delivery and adoption; it requires organisational change with a focus on introducing and incorporating the EHR into routine care by profession-als and/or patients within the healthcare organisation (Cresswell and Sheikh 2013). Governance, leadership and culture are all critical issues that influence the successful implementation and adoption of an EHR. It is important to appoint the right per-son to each leadership position at different levels of the organisation. The role of the nursing informatics specialist workforce was discussed in Chapter 5, and the role of leadership in digital transformation in Chapter 6. This chapter considers the specific organisational issues related to the implementation and adoption of an EHR.

There are different approaches to the implementation of EHRs, which will require different organisational change management and leadership strategies. One approach is that of a 'Big Bang', where the EHR is introduced at one point in time across all administrative and clinical services in the organisation. In contrast, phased implemen-tation of an EHR, also known as incremental or staggered implementation, may occur in various ways; for example, by hospital ward, class of data or function (e.g. prescrip-tions), locality (e.g. hospital group), type of care setting (e.g. acute hospitals), condi-tion or sub-population (e.g. maternity and newborn). There are risks and benefits to the two approaches. A 'Big Bang' is an example of extreme organisational change and disruption to services, which may have implications for the quality of service provi-sion in the short term, but may lead to acceptance of the system and higher adoption over time. Phased implementations have the risk of the organisation using a hybrid of paper and electronic charting at the same time. For example, in acute care, phased implementations often begin in in-patient settings, resulting in the transfer of many patient records from a paper-based emergency department to a ward using an EHR (Maguire et al. 2018). Choosing the most appropriate implementation approach for an organisation should be made based on individual requirements, resources and the change readiness of the stakeholders and organisation. One key consideration for the successful implementation of EHRs is collaborating with vendors, as it is important to ensure that there is a shared vision of success, and that they are open to sharing data and adapting the system to local needs (Maguire et al. 2018).

It is also important to nurture an organisational culture that is open to change, as implementation of an EHR is more of a clinical transformation project than an IT project. This requires involvement of all people who might be using the system in the planning, design and testing of the system, as well as supporting its implementation (Cresswell and Sheikh 2013). This is particularly important for nurses, who are the largest users of EHRs, and therefore have a significant impact on if, and how, an EHR is implemented. Having a culture that is open to shared learning, with effective communication and timely feedback is also supportive of effective change. Training the nurses who will be using the EHR is crucial to successful implementation and subsequent use of the system and can be carried out in a number of ways using strategies such as classroom-based task simulation, one-on-one via shadowing or supervision during clinical tasks, e-learning modules, paper-based manuals, group training sessions or different combinations of the above. Providing opportunities for nurses to learn and become familiar with the system and gaining practice outside of formal training has also been shown to help with EHR adoption (Amatayakul 2011).

Other factors at an organisational level that need to be considered include the level and type of support available to nurses during the go live phase as well as ongoing support, including both practical support in clinical areas and IT support. Besides a team of specialist digital nurses and training all nurses on the use of the EHR, having local champions or 'super-users' of the EHR system is also a strategy that is often used as a way of providing vital clinical support to nurses at the point of care (Nguyen et al. 2014). It is crucial that nurses across the organisation be involved in the customisation of an EHR to ensure that the system fits with clinical workflow (Kruse et al. 2016). However, this needs to be balanced with the unique opportunity the EHR provides to update current non-standardised practices, embed best practice standards and identify any inefficiencies and safety issues. In essence, there will need to be a modification of existing work practices to increase standardisation in routines and information flows. This needs to be managed to ensure benefits for nurses (such as having data for quality improvement and reduced documentation time).

LEARNING EXERCISE

List all the potential stakeholders that would use an EHR in your organisation. Carry out a SWOT analysis to identify where you think the strengths are in your organisation to support an EHR implementation, if there are any weaknesses or threats to successful implementation, and how you might maximise any opportunities. List the actions you could take to ensure that any digital implementation is successful in your organisation.

Human Factors

The people who use the system will determine if the adoption of an EHR by a healthcare organisation will be successful. Despite the organisational resources and structure, and the technology procured, individual skills and characteristics, as well as how the EHR affects their values and roles, will determine the acceptance and support of the system (Maguire et al. 2018).

As highlighted in Chapter 4, digital literacy is crucial to enable nurses to operate an EHR and change their attitudes towards adoption of the technology. Providing evidence of how the implementation of an EHR can benefit the delivery of nursing care, such as improved data quality, automation of mundane tasks and patient safety, can also significantly affect acceptance and successful use (Kruse et al. 2016). Ensuring that nurses involved in an EHR implementation understand there will be disruption in their ability to provide care and that there will be changes to work processes but that the benefits will be worthwhile, is crucial for success.

Technological Factors

The technology that nurses utilise will influence their overall satisfaction as well as the effectiveness and efficiency of how the EHR is used. Usability of a digital system refers to the ability of nurses to use the technology effectively to support their work practices. How usable an EHR is will influence how efficient nurses find the system, how much time they can spend with people, the quality of care they provide and patient safety. Most EHR systems are bought from vendors and will need to be customised to ensure the system is usable in the specific context where it is being deployed. If a system is not easy to use, nurses will develop 'workarounds'. For example, they may bypass some of the processes for ensuring patient safety (such as bar code scanning) or record vital signs on paper instead of entering them directly into the EHR (Fraczkowski et al. 2020). It is vital that nurses be part of the teams that test the EHR, including examining the clinical content and the work processes (clinical workflow) during the development phase. As highlighted in Chapters 5 and 6, nurses with a specialist knowledge of digital and the involvement of nurse leadership are crucial to ensuring that the EHR is usable.

Other factors that influence the usability of an EHR, and whether it can provide benefits to practicing nurses, include how well a system can share information between different types of technology infrastructure (known as interoperability). For example, when different digital systems are unable to share information in organisations (e.g. patient administration system unable to share data with medical imaging), it can lead to dual entry of information (which imposes a time burden on staff, including nurses) and poor communication. It can also lead to issues with patient safety. Ensuring that nurses have the infrastructure, including access to Wi-Fi, appropriate devices to access the EHR and systems in place to maintain that infrastructure is crucial for enabling successful EHR adoption.

Opportunities and Challenges

Implementing an EHR is only the beginning of an adoption process of a system that will require adaptation and further development to meet the changing needs of patient care (a process known as optimisation). Given the disruption it causes to the way in which care is provided across an organisation, and the impact it has on how nurses work, one can question whether implementing an EHR is worth the costs it involves. There are few studies that have evaluated the full benefits of EHR implementations; this is not surprising as EHRs comprise a number of different 'types' of technology, and an organisation (as highlighted previously) can choose to adopt some elements of an EHR (such as a medical imaging system) or have an organisation-wide integrated EHR. However, it is possible to evaluate the components that comprise an EHR and through this, identify some of the potential benefits for an organisation if an EHR is adopted successfully.

One study in Australia evaluated the effect of an EHR implementation on the amount of time nurses spent on different care tasks (Bingham et al. 2021). They found that after the EHR implementation, nurses spent less time on indirect care tasks and in carrying out 'in transit' activities (defined as time spent in between patients looking for equipment, other people or information) (Bingham et al. 2021). This study also found that nurses spent more time with patients and less time multitasking when carrying out a number of activities, including direct care, documentation and medication administration. Other studies have highlighted the positive impacts of introducing bar code medication administration on patient safety, including reducing medication administration errors (Shah et al. 2016).

However, as highlighted previously in this chapter, introducing EHRs can lead to a number of behaviours in nurses (known as workarounds) that may affect patient outcomes in unintended ways. These are often connected to systems that have poor usability (and therefore do not fit with nurses' workflows). Workarounds can lead to potentially negative outcomes for patient care (such as inaccurate vital signs documentation, transcription errors when taking data from paper and entering it into an electronic system) (Fraczkowski et al. 2020). Other studies have highlighted potential negative consequences for nurse/patient communication when using EHR technology. This includes anxiety that nurses' looking at a screen inhibits face-to-face communication and that there is a shift towards a more task-oriented formulaic approach to patient care (Forde-Johnson et al. 2023). However, the authors also highlight how strategies can be implemented to ensure a more patient-centred flexible approach to communication when using an EHR; the key is to acknowledge the potential impacts of an EHR and provide the training and environment to maximise the opportunities it provides.

LEARNING EXERCISE

Imagine you are in the process of implementing an EHR and you need to engage your nursing workforce in ensuring it is a success. List all the strategies you might use to achieve this – what challenges do you think you may face in your organisation? What might the eventual benefits be?

CASE STUDY

In 2015, Great Ormond Street Hospital for Children NHS Foundation Trust, a specialist paediatrics organisation, set a vision for its digital future, to introduce an electronic patient record (EPR). I was appointed as Chief Nursing Information Officer (CNIO) in January 2018, with the go live date set for just over a year later.

The EPR implementation was guided by three core values.

1. Patient welfare: Ensuring that the EPR implementation did not interfere with care safety.
2. Operational improvement: Ensuring the EPR helped us deliver care more efficiently.
3. Staff engagement: Clinicians needed to be part of the journey, helping us build efficient workflows.

Key steps I would recommend to any nursing colleague supporting a similar project.

- **Create a team:** Create a team of nursing informaticians with diverse backgrounds, skills and experience. This will produce an EPR tailored to the range of people in the organisation.
- **Learn from others:** Make friends and learn from national and international colleagues who have undertaken the journey before.
- **Review how care is provided:** Use the implementation as an opportunity to rethink care processes, and create new ways to provide care. EPR implementation is not only about digitising existing ways of working.
- **Take every opportunity to communicate with clinical colleagues about the implementation:** Invite yourself to every clinical meeting to talk about EPR and what it can mean for them.
- **Focus on change management:** There are challenges to leading a huge programme of change. The logistics of bringing an entire organisation on this journey at the same time as staff are facing normal day-to-day challenges were far from easy. Appoint change managers.
- **Get training right:** Familiarise staff with the system by giving them basic sessions on how it works and providing tip sheets. Recognise that you only really learn how to use an EPR when you actually start using it in practice.

I would also suggest running the implementation as though it were a major incident, enabling staff to bring any issues directly to the implementation team to either be actioned or to be provided support, and make EPR go live a celebration.

Implementing an EPR is one of the few times the whole organisation comes together to support a transformational change. It must be recognised that the true value is only seen later in opportunities to improve services and care delivery. One benefit is the availability of data. Using the data in the EPR, we have been able to create clinical dashboards, which have led to further standardisation and improvement in clinical workflows.

Conclusion

In this chapter, we provided an overview of the issues related to the successful implementation and adoption of EHRs and the importance of including nurses in the process. Introducing any digital technology will affect the way people work, and it is important to recognise that implementing an EHR is a transformation project. Nurse leadership at all levels of the organisation, and nurse engagement and involvement in the process of EHR adaptation and deployment, is critical for success.

Introducing an EHR can provide a number of opportunities to nurses and support care provision in a number of ways. This includes improved communication; reduced lack of time spent trying to find people, information, or equipment; and increased standardisation of routine practices. As discussed in other chapters in this book, with the provision of higher quality, standardised information located in an EHR, nurses can focus on improving care quality and using that information to inform research and care delivery. However, it is also important to recognise the challenges associated with EHR implementation and adoption. This includes recognising the potentially unintended consequences of using the technology for nurses' work, such as nurse/patient communication and how care is organised and delivered. Being aware of these challenges and putting strategies in place to ensure that nursing remains a person-centred practice can enable nurses to grasp the opportunities an EHR can provide to care delivery.

Key Points

1. Development and implementation of EHRs and other information technology offers significant opportunity to enhance nursing practice and the ability to evaluate and generate knowledge from nursing documentation.
2. Implementing an EHR requires organisational change to incorporate functionality into routine care.
3. An organisational culture that embraces change and strong nursing leadership are necessary to ensure successful implementation and adoption of an EHR.
4. The usability of an EHR will affect how it is used during the provision of nursing care. Nurses need to be involved in the development process to ensure the system integrates with workflow and supports their practice.
5. Introducing an EHR can improve care and patient safety; however, there needs to be recognition of the challenges it poses for person centred practice. Clear strategies need to be developed in the organisation to counteract this.

References

Amatayakul, M., 2011. Why workflow redesign alone is not enough for EHR success. Healthc. Financ. Manag. 65 (3), 130–132.

Bingham, G., Tong, E., Poole, S., et al., 2021. A longitudinal time and motion study quantifying how implementation of an electronic medical record influences hospital nurses' care delivery. Int. J. Med. Inf. 153, 104537. https://doi.org/10.1016/j.ijmedinf.2021.104537.

Cresswell, K., Sheikh, A., 2013. Organizational issues in the implementation and adoption of health information technology innovations: an interpretative review. Int. J. Med. Inf. 82 (5), e73–e86. https://doi.org/10.1016/j.ijmedinf.2012.10.007.

Forde-Johnston, C., Butcher, D., Aveyard, H., 2023. An integrative review exploring the impact of Electronic Health Records (EHR) on the quality of nurse–patient interactions and communication. J. Adv. Nurs. 79 (1), 48–67. https://doi.org/10.1111/jan.15484.

Fraczkowski, D., Matson, J., Lopez, K.D., 2020. Nurse workarounds in the electronic health record: an integrative review. J. Am. Med. Inf. Assoc. 27 (7), 1149–1165. https://doi.org/10.1093/jamia/ocaa050.

Kruse, C.S., Kristof, C., Jones, B., et al., 2016. Barriers to electronic health record adoption: a systematic literature review. J. Med. Syst. 40 (12), 252. https://doi.org/10.1007/s10916-016-0628-9.

Maguire, D., Evans, H., Honeyman, M., et al., 2018. Digital Change in Health and Social Care. The King's Fund, London.

Nguyen, L., Bellucci, E., Nguyen, L.T., 2014. Electronic health records implementation: an evaluation of information system impact and contingency factors. Int. J. Med. Inf. 83 (11), 779–796. https://doi.org/10.1016/j.ijmedinf.2014.06.011.

Shah, K., Lo, C., Babich, M., et al., 2016. Bar code medication administration technology: a systematic review of impact on patient safety when used with computerized prescriber order entry and automated dispensing devices. Can. J. Hosp. Pharm. 69 (5), 394–402. https://doi.org/10.4212/cjhp.v69i5.1594.

Clinical Decision Support

Dawn Dowding

Introduction

Worldwide, computerised clinical decision support systems (CDSS) are being integrated into digital technologies, such as electronic health records (EHRs). Typically, CDSS are designed to help support a clinician making decisions by bringing together information or characteristics of individuals being cared for, matched to a computerized clinical knowledge base. The system then provides individualised assessments or recommendations to the clinician, to help inform their decision making (Sutton et al. 2020).

The judgements and decisions taken by nurses have an impact on the quality and safety of patient care, as well as in the allocation of human and financial resources. For example, nurses assess people for their risk of developing pressure injuries and decide upon interventions (including allocation of specialist equipment) to prevent those injuries (Samuriwo et al. 2014). CDSS can help by providing up-to-date evidence-based information, making the process by which a decision is reached more explicit and consistent across healthcare professionals (Mebrahtu et al. 2021).

This chapter provides an overview of the different types of CDSS that nurses may encounter in their work. It also discusses research that explores the impact of CDSS on nurses' clinical practice, including patient safety, and provides insights into how different types of CDSS may impact how nurses think, depending on their experience and expertise. Finally, it discusses the role that nurses have in the development, implementation and use of CDSS across health and care settings.

TYPES OF CLINICAL DECISION SUPPORT SYSTEMS

There are a number of ways to classify the different types of CDSS nurses may come across in their clinical practice. One way of distinguishing between the different types of CDSS is to consider if they are 'knowledge based' or 'non-knowledge based' (Sutton et al. 2020). This classification refers to the type of clinical knowledge base that is accessed as part of the CDSS, with knowledge-based systems using decision rules (known as IF-THEN statements) to provide advice or guidance to the clinician. The decision rules can be derived from existing research evidence or systematic reviews, as well as knowledge of experts in the field (Sutton et al. 2020). In non-knowledge-based systems, large datasets (often taken from EHRs or other digital data sources) are analysed using statistical techniques, such as machine learning (often referred to as artificial intelligence or AI), to provide a recommendation to the clinician. With the growing availability of data, there has been an increasing focus on the development of AI-based decision support tools (O'Connor et al. 2022). However, there remain problems with their implementation, particularly in terms of the quality of the data used to inform the statistical algorithms and the lack of clarity regarding how an algorithm arrives at its decision recommendations. This implies that often, compared with the knowledge-based systems, clinicians and the people they care for do not trust the guidance provided by a decision support system that uses AI approaches (Young et al. 2021).

Other ways of classifying CDSS include approaches, such as when they are timed to occur in a decision process and whether they give decision support to a clinician regardless of whether they ask for it (active provision) or if they have to seek it out (passive support). A common approach is to classify different types of CDSS according to their function or the types of decisions they are designed to support. For example (Sutton et al. 2020) identified nine different types of CDSS according to their function, many of which are applicable to nursing practice (Table 9.1).

This highlights that there are many different types of CDSS, which have different aims and functions, and are often based on different types of knowledge base. Increasingly, diagnostics support for imaging, laboratory and pathology may be based on AI, whereas clinical management systems will often use knowledge-based approaches based on clinical guidelines and clinician expertise.

LEARNING EXERCISE

Using the information in Table 9.1, try to identify the CDSS that you currently use in your clinical practice (e.g. do you have a system you use to identify if a person's condition is deteriorating?). Do you know what type of knowledge it is based on? How do you think it affects the decisions you take when looking after people?

IMPACT OF CLINICAL DECISION SUPPORT ON NURSING PRACTICE

If nurses are going to use CDSS in their clinical practice, they need to be reassured that it will produce better outcomes for the people they look after or for

TABLE 9.1 ■ Types and Functions of Different Types of CDSS

Type of CDSS	Functions/Examples
Patient Safety	Reducing incidence of medication/prescribing errors and adverse events. Examples include computerised prescribing and bar code medication administration systems.
Clinical Management	Adherence to clinical guidelines, follow-up and treatment reminders.
Cost Containment	Reducing test and order duplication, suggesting cheaper medication or treatment options, automating administrative processes to reduce workload.
Administrative Function/Automation	Offering diagnostic code selection, automated documentation and note auto-fill.
Diagnostics Support	Providing diagnostic suggestions based on patient data, automating output from test results.
Diagnostics Support: Imaging, Laboratory and Pathology	Augmenting the extraction, visualisation and interpretation of medical images and laboratory test results.
Patient Decision Support	Decision support given to patients directly through personal health records and other systems.
Better Documentation	Consistency and accuracy of documentation electronically leads to improved decision making
Workflow Improvement	Improving the ability to retrieve and present data available in a person's clinical record in the EHR, resulting in the improvement and expedition of an existing workflow.

Adapted from Sutton et al. (2020).

their clinical care. One of the challenges with any intervention that tries to improve decision making in health and care environments is the inability to predict with certainty what a particular outcome may be. Therefore, to examine the effect CDSS may have on clinical practice, whether it encourages a more consistent process or whether a nurse has followed guidelines is evaluated, with the assumption that this will lead to better outcomes for the people being cared for.

In a systematic review of CDSS used by nurses, midwives and allied health professionals, (Mcbrahtu et al. 2021) identified 35 studies that evaluated the use of CDSS in clinical practice. The studies focused on five different types of outcomes related to the use of CDSS, including:

- Care processes, such as patient data collection and patient management
- Care outcomes, such as prevention of pressure ulcer
- Health professionals' knowledge, beliefs and behaviours, such as changes in attitudes due to the use of the CDSS

- Adverse events specifically related to patient safety
- Economic costs and consequences, such as cost savings or cost-effectiveness of the CDSS

Overall, the review found that using CDSS has the potential to improve care, with 26 (74.3%) of the included studies finding that care using CDSS was better than care without CDSS on at least one of the outcomes measured in the studies. For example, patients in emergency care being looked after by nurses using CDSS were more likely to have better blood glucose control; additionally, care processes, such as insulin dosing and blood sampling, at the right time were all better for nurses using CDSS (Mebrahtu et al. 2021).

The use of CDSS to support the prescribing and administration of medications is one area of clinical practice where there have been demonstrated improvements in the safety of care provided by nurses. For example, bar code medication administration systems (BCMA) include CDSS to ensure that the nurse is giving the right medication to the right patient at the right time (Shah et al. 2016). Evidence from a number of studies exploring the use of BCMA suggests that its use reduces errors in the administration of wrong dose, medication or route (Shah et al. 2016).

As highlighted previously, CDSS vary in their function and the types of decisions they support. The way in which they are designed to provide advice and guidance may also affect how they are used by clinicians, and consequently, the impact they have on practice. For example, (Van de Velde et al. 2018) suggest that if decision support advice is generated automatically and provided on a computer screen, it is more likely to be acted upon and have an impact on care processes.

EXPERTISE, DECISION MAKING AND CLINICAL DECISION SUPPORT

The main function of CDSS is to support clinicians, including nurses, in their decision making. However, how CDSS are used often vary depending on the experience and expertise of the individual using the system (Dowding et al. 2009). Typically, individuals who are less experienced in a clinical situation and those who do not have the background knowledge or expertise to help inform their decision making need to rely on rules, guidelines or protocols (Benner et al. 2009). In these situations, CDSS may help support their decision making by providing a clear pathway to follow, from obtaining information to reaching a decision.

In contrast, more experienced individuals who have expertise in an area and make decisions frequently are more likely to use fast, subconscious approaches to decision making (often referred to as intuition or a 'gut feeling'). For these individuals, the use of rule-based systems or protocols built into CDSS will be ineffective, as they feel they already 'know' what to do (Dowding et al. 2009). However, more experienced individuals may make some errors or mistakes in their decision making, as they are likely to use 'rules of thumb' or heuristics to inform their choices. For these individuals, CDSS that provide alerts to check if the individual really wants to choose a particular option (for example, a particular drug) or to suggest alternatives that may not have been considered, may be more effective.

LEARNING EXERCISE

Take one of the CDSS systems you have identified in your previous answer. Now, think about all the people you work with who use the system. Do different people use it differently? Why do think that might be?

As discussed in Chapter 8 in this book, a significant body of research indicates that if CDSS (as well as other types of digital technology) are not designed to take into account nurses' clinical workflow (including the information used and how they carry out their work) when they are designed, then users (in this case nurses) will figure out a way to 'work around' the CDSS processes. For example, nurses have been found to integrate knowledge from CDSS into their practice, meaning that they do not use CDSS guidance when taking decisions, manipulate the algorithms in CDSS to provide the 'right' answer, and are more likely to override CDSS recommendations if they are more experienced (Dowding et al. 2009). A systematic review of nurses' workarounds when using EHR systems identified 8 different types of workarounds, incorporating 36 different types of behaviours, implying that the system was not used as it was designed (Fraczkowski et al. 2020). Whilst EHRs are not the same as CDSS, many of the workarounds identified in the review have implications for the effectiveness of CDSS or are related to specific CDSS inbuilt into the EHR.

Figure. 9.1 provides a summary of the workaround strategies and behaviours. Examples of the relevance of these workarounds for CDSS include:

- Using paper as a cognitive tool – documenting on paper and then entering data into the EHR at a later date means that any CDSS that relies on accurate and timely data to provide decision recommendations or alerts will not be reliable. For example, alert systems that use vital signs information to indicate if a patient is deteriorating rely on timely, accurate vital signs information being recorded in the EHR.
- Bypassing patient identification or EHR medication checks – any CDSS associated with checking the patient, medication, dose and time will not be triggered in a timely fashion. The checks are designed to ensure that alerts regarding safety of medication administration occur *before* a medication is administered to the patient. If checks are bypassed, then this will not happen.

THE ROLE OF NURSES IN CLINICAL DECISION SUPPORT

With the growing acceleration of the use of digital technology in health and care settings, nurses will increasingly use CDSS (either knowingly or unknowingly) in their clinical practice. As highlighted in the previous section, if digital technology

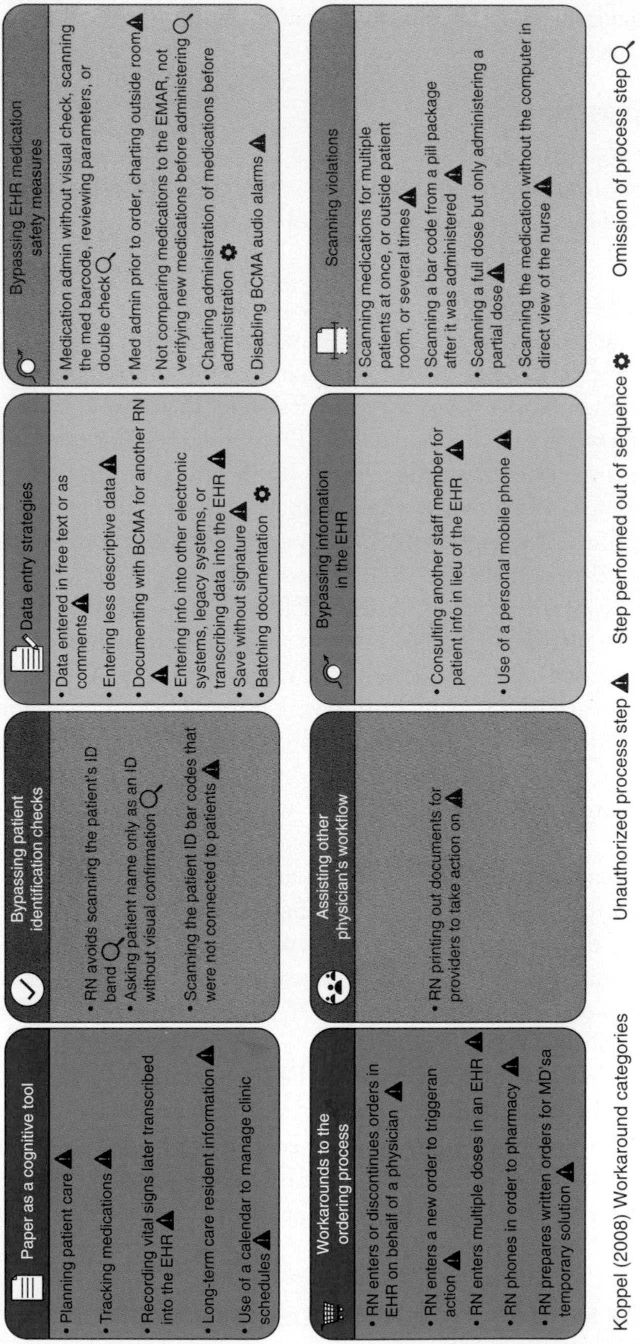

Paper as a cognitive tool
- Planning patient care ▲
- Tracking medications ▲
- Recording vital signs later transcribed into the EHR ▲
- Long-term care resident information ▲
- Use of a calendar to manage clinic schedules ▲

Bypassing patient identification checks
- RN avoids scanning the patient's ID band ◯
- Asking patient name only as an ID without visual confirmation ◯
- Scanning the patient ID bar codes that were not connected to patients ▲

Data entry strategies
- Data entered in free text or as comments ▲
- Entering less descriptive data ▲
- Documenting with BCMA for another RN ▲
- Entering info into other electronic systems, legacy systems, or transcribing data into the EHR ▲
- Save without signature ▲
- Batching documentation ✿

Bypassing EHR medication safety measures
- Medication admin without visual check, scanning the med barcode, reviewing parameters, or double check ◯
- Med admin prior to order, charting outside room ▲
- Not comparing medications to the EMAR, not verifying new medications before administering ◯
- Charting administration of medications before administration ✿
- Disabling BCMA audio alarms ▲

Workarounds to the ordering process
- RN enters or discontinues orders in EHR on behalf of a physician ▲
- RN enters a new order to trigger an action ▲
- RN enters multiple doses in an EHR ▲
- RN phones in order to pharmacy ▲
- RN prepares written orders for MD's a temporary solution ▲

Assisting other physician's workflow
- RN printing out documents for providers to take action on ▲

Bypassing information in the EHR
- Consulting another staff member for patient info in lieu of the EHR ▲
- Use of a personal mobile phone ▲

Scanning violations
- Scanning medications for multiple patients at once, or outside patient room, or several times ▲
- Scanning a bar code from a pill package after it was administered ▲
- Scanning a full dose but only administering a partial dose ▲
- Scanning the medication without the computer in direct view of the nurse ▲

Koppel (2008) Workaround categories   Unauthorized process step ▲   Step performed out of sequence ✿   Omission of process step ◯

Fig. 9.1   Registered nurse workaround strategies and behaviours (Adapted from Fraczkowski et al. 2020)

systems, including CDSS, are not designed in collaboration with the users of the systems, they may not be used in a way that leads to effective healthcare practice. This means that nurses have an important role to play in the development, implementation and use of CDSS.

When CDSS are being developed and if nurses are the target users of the system, then they should have a key role in helping inform the process. At present, nurses are often not a part of the teams that develop or implement CDSS. For example, (O'Connor et al. 2022) found that of the 140 studies that reported on the development or implementation of AI-based systems, only 41 (29.3%) had a nurse leading the research and 9 (6.42%) involved nurses in the active checking of the models used in the AI system. In nearly half of the studies (68 or 48.6%), nurses were not involved in the AI development, implementation or evaluation. If nurses are involved in the process, then the likelihood of workarounds when using systems such as CDSS will be reduced.

CASE STUDY

NEWS is a tool developed by the Royal College of Physicians which supports practitioners in detecting and responding to clinical deterioration in adult patients and is a key element of patient safety and improving patient outcomes.

The tool is based on a scoring system, in which a score is allocated to physiological measurements already recorded in routine practice. Six physiological parameters form the basis of the scoring system and are used to provide an aggregated score, which is then used to provide guidance to the staff on actions needed to support good patient outcomes. This standardised approach can reduce the number of patients whose conditions deteriorate whilst in hospital and can potentially save over 1800 lives a year.

The senior nursing team at Imperial College Healthcare NHS Trust identified that the existing paper-based approach to documentation of a patient's observations was varied across the Trust, and a robust tool to identify deterioration which could contribute to patient safety incidents was not standardized practice. To address this unwarranted variation, the 'Safer Care Project' was initiated at the Trust using digital technology to identify patients at risk of deterioration and to provide optimal care to improve their outcomes and experience.

Handheld devices were introduced to reduce documentation time with decision support at the bedside. Digital touch screen monitors capture clinical observations such as blood pressure and temperature and automatically transfer it to the electronic patient record (EPR) via wireless connection. The EPR is supported by a handover page detailing a patient's latest NEWS score that is automatically calculated, and any escalation instructions automatically appear on screen.

Introducing the system has led to improvements in patient safety. The mean time to take and record vitals has reduced and by using bedside devices, 600 hours of nursing time has been released from routine documentation, time that can be used in direct patient care.

Adapted from NHS England 2019.

Conclusion

This chapter provided an overview of the main types of CDSS used in healthcare practice. It highlighted the range of different types of CDSS that may be available to nurses in their clinical practice, including the types of knowledge-base used for the CDSS as well as the types of functions or decisions that they can support. It is important for nurses to understand the role and function of CDSS when they are implemented in health and care settings. By understanding the nature and function of CDSS, they can evaluate if and how it is being used in their practice, and highlight areas where systems could be improved, or workarounds explored to ensure that the CDSS are used to help improve care.

With the increasing development of non-knowledge-based CDSS, such as systems based on AI algorithms across the health and care sector, it is likely that the implementation of such approaches will increase in the future. Understanding the implications of this for nursing practice is important in terms of the data collected and used to inform AI and CDSS, as well as in terms of also how that may impact on the way nurses work. There are opportunities for nurses to become partners in the development and implementation of CDSS, and with the increasing role of nursing informatics professionals in healthcare settings, to ensure that decisions taken about systems fully involve nurses in the decision process.

Key Points

1. CDSS can be classified as 'knowledge-based' or 'non-knowledge-based' systems, depending on whether the information they use to provide decision guidance comes from research evidence, expert opinion, or statistical analysis of large datasets.
2. CDSS vary significantly and can provide a number of functions, such as improving adherence to clinical guidelines and reducing the number of errors made during clinical care. Evidence suggests that using CDSS improves care outcomes and reduces patient safety events.
3. How CDSS are used in health and care practices varies depending on the experience or expertise of the nurses using the system. It is important to understand the type of CDSS that is being implemented in a practice setting and who the target users are, to provide the 'best match' between user and CDSS.
4. If nurses are not involved in the design and implementation of CDSS, then the system is more likely to not fit with how they work. This in turn may lead to 'workarounds', which may lead to CDSS not being effective in supporting decision making in health and care settings.
5. Ensuring that nurses have an overview of the CDSS' aim, understand who will be expected to use it and how it has been developed, as well as ensuring that nurses are included in the process of development, implementation and evaluation has the potential to lead to improved care.

References

Benner, P.E., Chesla, C.A., Tanner, C.A., 2009. Expertise in Nursing Practice: Caring, Clinical Judgment & Ethics. Springer, New York.

Dowding, D., Randell, R., Mitchell, N., et al., 2009. Experience and nurses use of computerised decision support systems. Stud. Health Technol. Inform. 146, 506–510.

Fraczkowski, D., Matson, J., Lopez, K.D., 2020. Nurse workarounds in the electronic health record: an integrative review. J. Am. Med. Inform. Assoc. 27 (7), 1149–1165. https://doi.org/10.1093/jamia/ocaa050.

Mebrahtu, T.F., Skyrme, S., Randell, R., et al., 2021. Effects of computerised Clinical Decision Support Systems (CDSS) on nursing and allied health professional performance and patient outcomes: a systematic review of experimental and observational studies. BMJ Open 11 (12), e053886. https://doi.org/10.1136/bmjopen-2021-053886.

NHS England, 2019. Introducing bedside vital signs devices at Imperial College Healthcare NHS Trust. Available at: https://www.england.nhs.uk/atlas_case_study/introducing-bedside-vital-signs-devices-at-imperial-college-healthcare-nhs-trust/.

O'Connor, S., Yan, Y., Thilo, F.J.S., et al., 2022. Artificial intelligence in nursing and midwifery: a systematic review. J. Clin. Nurs. https://doi.org/10.1111/jocn.16478.

Samuriwo, R., Dowding, D., 2014. Nurses' pressure ulcer related judgements and decisions in clinical practice: a systematic review. Int. J. Nurs. Stud. 51 (12), 1667–1685. https://doi.org/10.1016/j.ijnurstu.2014.04.009.

Shah, K., Lo, C., Babich, M., et al., 2016. Bar code medication administration technology: a systematic review of impact on patient safety when used with computerized prescriber order entry and automated dispensing devices. Can. J. Hosp. Pharm. 69 (5), 394–402. https://doi.org/10.4212/cjhp.v69i5.1594.

Sutton, R.T., Pincock, D., Baumgart, D.C., et al., 2020. An overview of clinical decision support systems: benefits, risks, and strategies for success. NPJ Digit. Med. 3, 17. https://doi.org/10.1038/s41746-020-0221-y.

Van de Velde, S., Heselmans, A., Delvaux, N., et al., 2018. A systematic review of trials evaluating success factors of interventions with computerised clinical decision support. Implement. Sci. 13 (1), 114. https://doi.org/10.1186/s13012-018-0790-1.

Young, A.T., Amara, D., Bhattacharya, A., et al., 2021. Patient and general public attitudes towards clinical artificial intelligence: a mixed methods systematic review. Lancet Digit. Health. 3 (9), e599–e611. https://doi.org/10.1016/S2589-7500(21)00132-1.

CHAPTER 10

Creating a Digital Clinical Safety Culture

Holly Carr

Introduction

On 4 November 1854, a young 'sick' nurse arrived off the coast of Scutari, Turkey and set a course that would change the landscape of healthcare forever. Patient safety has been a cornerstone of nursing practice since the exceptional work of nurse and statistician Florence Nightingale during the Crimean War. Safety underpins every decision nurses make, maintaining the wellbeing of their patients and preventing harm during the provision of care. Many would describe it as the 'art of nursing'. However, how can nurses ensure that they continue to cultivate and maintain this superpower in a digital world?

This chapter reflects on the history and evolution of patient safety in a digital world, exploring the barriers and enablers to instilling a positive culture of digital clinical safety across health and care and highlighting why the nursing profession is so well placed to lead this agenda.

A BRIEF HISTORY OF PATIENT SAFETY

It is hard to believe that patient safety was not always at the epicentre of healthcare provision and quality improvement. Whilst the Lady with the Lamp, Florence

Nightingale, pioneered the use of data to drive better patient outcomes, patient safety was not established as a standalone concept, nor did it garner national attention until the ground-breaking report 'To Err is Human: Building a safer Health System' was published by the US Institute of Medicine (IOM) in 2000. The report, which examined the consequences of medical errors across healthcare, estimated that a staggering 44,000–98,000 deaths were preventable per year across American hospitals. The jarring statistic, which was equated to a jumbo jet full of passengers crashing every 36 hours, galvanised an international campaign that not only established the standalone field of patient safety but also redefined the concept of quality improvement (Leape 2021).

The years following the revolutionary publication witnessed substantial efforts being made to identify sources of errors, develop safety metrics and create impactful strategy, policy and guidance to improve safety across all areas of health and care. In 2000, a seminal report titled 'An Organisation with Memory' advocated for the modernisation of the national approach to safety in the United Kingdom, focusing on centralised reporting and analysis to identify and learn from incidents in the hope of preventing subsequent failures (Department of Health 2000). Metrics to define and measure 'preventable harm' have subsequently moved beyond mortality to consider the holistic impact on a persons' morbidity, prognosis, quality of life and loss of dignity; this approach considers the patient as a whole and redefines the parameters of error.

Whilst the impact of reporting on the field of patient safety is undeniable, the global movement towards a safer healthcare system also prompted significant developments in the universal approach to quality improvement. The inclusion of safety as a pillar of quality, that is, the expansion of quality to include safety in various frameworks and definitions, has influenced an approach of learning from what went well and led to the rise of a safety conscious culture in healthcare. Whilst there have been marked improvements across focused areas of patient safety in the past 22 years, progress has been relatively slow and improving patient safety in healthcare continues to remain a pressing global priority (Flott et al. 2018).

CLINICAL SAFETY IN A DIGITAL WORLD

Since March 2019, there has been a marked increase in the uptake and adoption of digital technologies across health and care systems internationally, as ways of working changed in response to the Covid-19 pandemic, irreversibly altering the landscape of both digital health and patient safety. Prior to the pandemic, an estimated 80% of primary care appointments in England were face-to-face. By June 2020, this significantly reduced to below 50% as the use of digital technology in the National Health Service increased by 38% (Horton et al. 2021). The introduction of new technologies, such as remote monitoring, virtual wards and virtual consultations, truly demonstrates the opportunity for digital technology to liberate innovation and redefine what it means to deliver patient centred care.

Whilst evidence acknowledges the intrinsic ability of digital technologies to support and improve safer care, mounting evidence suggests a potential for increased risk and potential disruption (NHS Transformation Directorate 2021). Digital clinical safety refers to the avoidance of harm to patients and staff as a result of technologies manufactured, implemented and used in the health service. Safety is not a static concept, but is one that is fluid and responsive to the changing needs of health services, patients and citizens in response to new and emerging risks. Accelerations, such as the pandemic, have prompted a renewed emphasis on ensuring digital health technologies' safety, both in their design and implementation.

Whilst the drive to promptly identify and report risks and incidents relating to digital clinical safety has resulted in increased cataloguing of harm, it is widely recognised that an honest and open culture, person-centred design and innovation are key to reducing incidence of error; in essence, creating a positive digital clinical safety culture (Lark et al. 2018).

CREATING A POSITIVE DIGITAL CLINICAL SAFETY CULTURE

A safety culture is defined as a culmination of individual and group values, attitudes, perceptions, competencies, and patterns of behaviour that determine the commitment to, and the style and proficiency of an organisation's approach to health and safety management. Organisations that practice a 'good' safety culture often exhibit similar characteristics, with a shared understanding and perception of the importance of safety, consistently open communication with trust and impactful processes to identify and mitigate risks and incidents.

Healthcare is dynamic and disparate, with significant variation across healthcare settings, specialisms, provider organisations and patient groups, contributing to vastly different and unique organisational cultures (Lark et al. 2018). One size does not fit all, and a multi-faceted approach, including national standards and guidance, localised identification and reporting processes, workforce education, communication and safety centric design, is required to stabilise the foundations on which to cultivate a positive digital clinical safety culture across health and care.

STANDARDS AND GUIDANCE

Whilst accountability for the safety of a system rests with system providers and local organisations, the authority on requirements surrounding digital clinical safety is typically upheld by law and national regulations, which ensure intrinsic safety of digital technologies used within healthcare settings.

In England, clinical risk management standards (Table 10.1), mandated for use under the Health and Care Act 2012, outline specifications and guidance.

Clinical risk management standards exist within a wider network of regulations, such as cyber security and information governance, to ensure that both suppliers

TABLE 10.1 ■ **Clinical Risk Management Standards in England**

Standards	Specifications
DCB0129	This standard applies to the manufacturers of IT systems and outlines a set of requirements to promote and ensure the effective application of clinical risk management by providers and organisations responsible for the design, development, and maintenance of digital health systems.
DCB0160	This standard applies to the healthcare organisations implementing IT systems and outlines a set of requirements to promote and ensure the effective application of clinical risk management by organisations responsible for the deployment, use, maintenance and decommissioning of digital health systems.
Digital Technology Assessment Criteria (DTAC)	This assessment criteria are designed to be used by healthcare organisations to assess suppliers at the point of procurement or as part of a due diligence process to ensure that digital technologies meet clinical safety, data protection, technical security, interoperability, usability and accessibility standards.

and local providers perform due diligence when it comes to considering adequate risk mitigation during system development, design, implementation and decommission. Whilst they provide a foundation on which to build a positive safety culture, lack of regulation and loose interpretation often inhibits reliable implementation. Examples of best practice and shared learning can facilitate further contextualisation and greater understanding. However, unless digital clinical safety becomes a universal language and shared responsibility, the struggle to balance opportunity and risk will continue.

LEARNING EXERCISE

Reflect on the following scenarios and identify which clinical risk management standard applies:
1. Your organisation is entering a commercial procurement process and you would like to ensure that correct measures have been taken by the system provider to ensure the safety of their product. What would you request to see from the system provider and which national standard would you assess the supplier against?
2. Your organisation has decided to implement a 'home grown' electronic patient record. Which standards must you adhere to throughout the design and implementation process?

EDUCATION AND TRAINING

How do we ensure the technology we are using is safe? How can we optimise ways of working using digital technology to promote safter care and innovation? How can we assure the correct identification of digital clinical safety risks and incidents and identify mitigations?

A positive digital clinical safety culture needs to be championed from ward to board. What was once deemed the sole responsibility of colleagues working in technology is now shared amongst the wider healthcare workforce and should be a priority for anyone involved either directly or indirectly in patient care. This requires a foundation of knowledge and a language that speaks to both the technical and clinical elements, enabling interpretation of standards and guidance from a leadership perspective and risk and issue identification from a user perspective.

The person facing workforce needs to have the language and knowledge to not only be able to identify patient safety risks, near misses and incidents, but also articulate these in a way that is impactful and resonates with those who design and configure the systems. Digital systems should not define the way nurses care for people but rather better support clinical decisions and enable new ways of working.

There is widespread, deep-rooted hesitancy around the use of digital technology in healthcare, and the 'not my responsibility' mentality that goes alongside this opens the door to potential misuse. There is a tendency to see digital as a departure from the 'norm' and something that should only be used by those who are 'tech savvy' or of a 'younger generation', when in fact digital clinical safety relates to long established ways of working as well as new practices and processes.

IDENTIFICATION AND REPORTING

Errors, incidents and accidents across all healthcare settings have the capacity to cause serious harm to patients (Lark et al. 2018). To encourage a positive safety culture, learning from and understanding when and why things go wrong are crucial to prevent it from happening again.

Whilst local cataloguing of incidents has been embedded for some time to inform organisational strategy and priorities, there is recognition that a centralised reporting system could support further advances in tackling tenacious clinical safety issues, particularly where digital technology is concerned (NHS Transformation Directorate, n.d.). In England, the National Reporting and Learning System (NRLS) was introduced by the National Patient Safety Agency to collate data on patient safety incidents. The data is analysed to identify hazards, risks, incidents and opportunities to improve the safety of patient care, with findings being disseminated to local organisations. This data can also be used to inform national strategy, policy and decision-making.

In order to predict the impact of potential digital clinical safety issues and to mitigate those issues, it is important to first understand the interchangeable relationship between hazards, risks and incidents (Fig. 10.1).

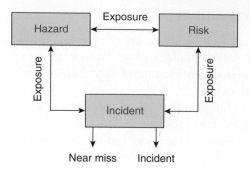

Fig. 10.1   The relationship between hazards, risks and incidents

TABLE 10.2 ■ Classification of Near Misses and Incidents

Classification	Definition
No harm	Any incident encountered that had the potential to cause harm but was prevented, resulting in no harm, or occurred but resulted in no harm.
Low	Any incident that required additional observation or minor treatment and caused minimal harm to the person involved.
Moderate	Any incident that resulted in a moderate increase in treatment and which caused significant but not permanent harm to the person involved.
Severe	Any incident that appears to have resulted in permanent harm to an individual or multiple persons.
Death	Any incident that directly resulted in the death of one or more persons.

We define hazards as a situation or condition that has the potential to cause harm (e.g. *two patients with the same name are placed in the same bay on a busy ward*). A risk is the probability of an incident occurring measured alongside the predicted severity of an outcome if an incident were to happen (e.g. *both patients are due to have their clinical observations at 10:00. Patient A has a chronic condition and Patient B is usually fit and well*). A patient safety incident is defined as an unexpected or unintended episode which has the potential to, or resulted in, harm to the patient (e.g. *at 10:00, both Patient A and Patient B have a set of observations completed and documented without confirmation of identification. Patient B has deteriorated; however, his observations were recorded in Patient A's record. As a result, it did not trigger an escalation. Consequently, Patient B's condition continued to deteriorate without intervention*).

The classification and grading of near misses and incidents inform a mitigation or intervention proportionate to the risk of harm encountered, instilling appropriate safety interventions whilst also preventing it from happening again in the future (Table 10.2).

SAFETY BY DESIGN

Whilst digital health systems have an innate ability to reduce instances of human error, there is still potential for unanticipated malfunction and unintended mistakes. Digital transformation is not about digital at all, but rather people and processes; the transformation and optimisation of care pathways supported by the use of digital technology.

Oversight in user-centred design can lead to an increase in patient safety risks and incidents and result in a system that is ultimately not fit for the purpose. After all, technology is not a substitute for the care provided, but rather a vehicle to support clinical decision-making and to better connect the care surrounding the patient.

Digital clinical safety is often an afterthought or a last-minute tick box exercise within the digital transformation journey. This frequently results in frustration, delays in implementation and conflict. By embedding a safety-by-design approach that instils rigorous safety governance processes, clinical engagement, clinical optimisation of care pathways and a patient-centred design from procurement to implementation, reduces the risk of creating a system that is riddled with potential safety risks and does not meet the needs of patients and those caring for them.

LEARNING EXERCISE

Read the case study above and consider the following:
1. What do you think went well and contributed to the success of the digital clinical safety project?
2. What was tricky?
3. What could be done differently next time?
4. What are some of the cultural challenges you would face within your organisation if you conducted a similar project?

CASE STUDY: NURSE-LED DIGITAL CLINICAL SAFETY (PAM FEARNS – DIGITAL MATRON)

When planning any digital implementation, it is essential to have a clear understanding of the impact on clinicians and workflows, but more importantly, of any potential safety risks for the patient.

As a Digital Nurse Implementer, I was involved the design and implementation of a web-based application that used messaging and alerts on a phone, tablet or a desktop device, to replace the existing bleep system.

During the configuration phase, current workflows were mapped and optimised with input from clinicians, nurses and the clinical digital team. This ensured that the new system did not pose a safety risk and had all the required functionality. A multidisciplinary pilot group was established to rigorously test the new process, including a specified ward area, Speciality Registrars, and the Critical Care Outreach Team.

During the pilot, the new application was trialled alongside the existing bleep system. It could be argued that this discouraged the uptake of the new application, as staff often revert to what they know, particularly when they are busy. However, the alternative would have been to remove the existing bleeps for the pilot group, which

CASE STUDY: NURSE-LED DIGITAL CLINICAL SAFETY (PAM FEARNS – DIGITAL MATRON)—cont'd

could have inadvertently created unforeseen clinical risks. Following limited uptake during the initial pilot, a second group of clinicians were engaged, and the pilot scaled.

My role within the project team was to engage clinical staff, promote uptake of the system, highlight its benefits and listen to feedback at the point of care. Several issues were raised during the pilot, were logged within a hazard log and escalated to developers using a priority and impact matrix, which prompted quick turnaround of fixes. This resulted in a system that met the needs of the clinicians and patients. Show-and-tell sessions were set up to showcase the application, but we also attended the clinical areas on numerous occasions, over several weeks, to capture staff on different shifts and train them to use the application before the Go-Live date.

Following this project, I have reflected on what went well, what was difficult and what I would do differently. Being a visible presence throughout the pilot was vital to capturing as many staff as possible for training and to gaining feedback and addressing issues raised in a prompt manner. Having different forums to engage and train all staff groups, including online drop-in sessions, one-on-ones and group sessions in the clinical areas was also pivotal, as different staff groups and specialties had different training requirements. Changing the culture was challenging, with one of the biggest difficulties being promoting the benefits of the new system when some staff felt what they had was perfectly adequate. My main takeaway from this project is to keep reflecting throughout the end-to-end process and to adapt your approach accordingly.

Conclusion

Hopefully by this stage, you have a good understanding of what it takes to build and sustain a positive digital clinical safety culture within your organisation. However, you may also be left wondering, 'why me?'.

As the most trusted profession, nurses hold the hand of the patient throughout their entire healthcare journey, coming into contact at each stage of intervention and coordinating with the wider multi-disciplinary team around the patients care pathway. Due to the nature of their work, nurses play a pivotal role in maintaining and promoting a culture of digital clinical safety and clinical risk management.

Safety has always been a cornerstone of nursing practice. As the largest workforce operating across all areas of health and social care, being the primary deliverers of direct patient care and the predominant handlers of both technology and data, nurses are best placed to safeguard and advocate for the needs of their patients and multi-disciplinary colleagues, driving a culture of digital clinical safety.

This chapter explored the origins and evolution of patient safety in a digital world and highlighted the pivotal role nurses play in leading and championing a culture of digital clinical safety. It explored the fundamental components of building and sustaining a positive digital clinical safety culture and provided a series of practical hints and tips to consider in nurses' day-to-day practice to ensure patient safety remains at the forefront of the technology-enabled care provided.

Key Points

1. Patient safety is a key issue of quality measurement for healthcare organisations internationally.
2. Substantial efforts have been made to identify sources of error, develop safety metrics, and create impactful strategy, policy and guidance to improve safety across all areas of health and care.
3. Working alongside clinical teams in their organisation to visualise and optimise ways of working before configuring and building within the digital system can ensure that the implementation is right the first time and that the appropriate safety considerations are adequately captured and mitigated within the system.
4. Working alongside Clinical Safety Officer to embed digital clinical safety process throughout the digital transformation process and not as an afterthought or a tick box exercise prior to going live is crucial.
5. Digital clinical safety standards compliance should be included within the procurement specification. Suppliers should be asked for their clinical safety case reports.

References

Department of Health, 2000. An Organisation with a Memory: Report of an Expert Group on Learning from Adverse Events in the NHS. The Stationery Office, London.

Flott K, Durkin M, Darzi A. (2108) The Tokyo Declaration on patient safety. BMJ 362:k3424. https://doi.org/10.1136/bmj.k34240

Horton, T., Hardie, T., Mahadeva, S., et al., 2021. Securing a Positive Health Care Technology Legacy from COVID-19. Health Foundation. Available at: https://www.health.org.uk/publications/long-reads/securing-a-positive-health-care-technology-legacy-from-covid-19.

Institute of Medicine (US), 2002. Committee on quality of health care in America. In: Kohn, L.T., Corrigan, J.M., Donaldson, M.S. (Eds.), To Err Is Human: Building a Safer Health System. National Academies Press, Washington (DC).

Lark, M.E., Kirkpatrick, K., Chung, K.C., 2018. Patient safety movement: history and future directions. J. Hand Surg. 43 (2), 174–178. https://doi.org10.1016/j.jhsa.2017.11.006.

Leape, L., 2021. Making Healthcare Safe: The story of the Patient Safety Movement. Springer, Switzerland.

NHS Transformation Directorate, 2021. Digital Clinical Safety Strategy. Available at: https://transform.england.nhs.uk/key-tools-and-info/digital-clinical-safety-strategy/.

Further reading

Patient Safety Learning – the hub. (n.d.). (200) An organisation with a memory. Available at: https://www.pslhub.org/learn/organisations-linked-to-patient-safety-uk-and-beyond/government-and-alb-direction-and-guidance/dhsc/an-organisation-with-a-memory-june-2000-r1380/.

Schiff, G., Shojania, K.G., 2021. Looking back on the history of patient safety: an opportunity to reflect and ponder future challenges. BMJ Quality & Safety 31 (2), 148–152. https://doi.org/10.1136/bmjqs-2021-014163.

NHS Transformation Directorate. (n.d.). Digital Technology Assessment Criteria (DTAC). Available at: https://transform.england.nhs.uk/key-tools-and-info/digital-technology-assessment-criteria-dtac/.

NHS Digital. (n.d.). DCB0160: Clinical risk management: its application in the deployment and use of health IT systems. Available at: https://digital.nhs.uk/data-and-information/information-standards/information-standards-and-data-collections-including-extractions/publications-and-notifications/standards-and-collections/dcb0160-clinical-risk-management-its-application-in-the-deployment-and-use-of-health-it-systems.

NHS Digital. (n.d.). DCB0129: Clinical risk management: its application in the manufacture ofhealthITsystems.Availableat:https://digital.nhs.uk/data-and-information/information-standards/information-standards-and-data-collections-including-extractions/publications-and-notifications/standards-and-collections/dcb0129-clinical-risk-management-its-application-in-the-manufacture-of-health-it-systems.

Flott, K., Maguire, J., Phillips, N., 2021. Digital safety: the next frontier for patient safety. Future Healthcare Journal 8 (3), e598–e601. https://doi.org/10.7861/fhj.2021-0152.

CHAPTER 11

Information Governance and Cyber Security

Jo Dickson

LEARNING OUTCOMES

At the end of this chapter, the nurses will be able to:

- Identify examples of information governance relevant to health and social care, including principles governing confidentiality, information sharing, data protection, freedom of information rights and subject access requests.
- Evaluate their own practice of confidentiality and data protection.
- Develop an awareness of the management, economic, legal, social, professional and ethical issues relating to cyber security for health and care.

Introduction

The last 30 years have witnessed an explosion in the volume of information created and used within health and care services. The development of new technology has opened many new possibilities for the use of data to revolutionise care and significantly improve clinical outcomes. However, this increase has opened new and previously unimagined risks of information misuse. Organisations of all sizes are vulnerable to risks along a continuum from individual error to large-scale cyber-attack.

As discussed in Chapter 8, sharing relevant information at the right time is important, as is a perceived benefit of introducing digital systems, such as electronic patient records (EPRs). It can help nurses make informed decisions, ensuring that people receive safe care, enabling the smooth transition of people between different care settings and enhancing the effectiveness and efficiency of the service (Ham et al. 2018).

Information Governance (IG) is a strategic framework consisting of the standards, processes, roles and criteria used by organisations and systems for creating, organising, securing, preserving, using and disclosing/disseminating information. Cyber security is a subcomponent of IG; specifically, protecting electronic information from unauthorized access, use and disclosure. There are three goals of cyber security: protecting the confidentiality, integrity and availability of information.

Although different countries provide different health and care services to their citizens, any health system is expected to provide quality care for individuals, maintain community health, reduce per capita healthcare costs and adopt the best policies and decisions based on valid information. This chapter increases the knowledge of IG and cyber security and supplies nurses with tools and techniques to ensure safe and effective use of information in their practice.

INFORMATION GOVERNANCE

IG encompasses more than traditional data and records management. It incorporates information security and protection, compliance, data quality, data governance, risk management, privacy, data storage and archiving, analytics and data science.

Of all industry sectors, healthcare probably has the most intensive focus on IG. It is not hard to see why. The effective use of information is vital for good patient care and effective treatment. Patients and citizens expect that healthcare professionals manage and use data or information that identifies them appropriately. Thus, healthcare professionals should ensure the same standards they would expect when managing their own personal and sensitive information to be used by all those who work in health and social care settings.

Within a healthcare organisation, IG is the framework of standards for handling information in a confidential and secure manner. It provides guidelines on how to deal with service user/patients and employees' information, especially when that information is personal and sensitive. IG regulations are often set at a regulatory level within a country. It is therefore key that nurses understand the requirements within their own country. For example, in the United States, requirements are set by the Health Insurance Portability and Accountability Act (HIPAA) and in the UK by the EU General Data Protection Regulation (GDPR) and the UK Data Protection Act (2018).

All health and care organisations have a designated individual at the executive level who is accountable for upholding relevant legislation, as well as for ensuring policies are in place and audited against. They are also accountable for ensuring that suitable training is provided to all staff and that they are given time to complete said training. It is important that departmental and service leads understand their own responsibilities in this area, utilising the policies and tools provided by the organisation and supporting continuous improvement and learning from incidents.

BASIC PRINCIPLES OF INFORMATION GOVERNANCE

Information should be:
- used fairly, lawfully and transparently
- used for specified, explicit purposes
- used in a way that is adequate, relevant and limited to only what is necessary
- accurate and where necessary kept up to date
- kept for no longer than is necessary

- handled in a way that ensures appropriate security, including protection against unlawful or unauthorised processing, loss, destruction or damage.

(Royal College of Nursing 2022)

INFORMATION SHARING

Health and care professionals have a legal duty to share information to support the care of an individual. This is supported by law and in the UK, by a set of principles known as the Caldicott Principles. These principles apply to the use of confidential information within health and social care organisations and for when such information is shared with other organisations and between individuals, both for individual care and for other purposes.

The principles are intended to apply to all data collected for the provision of health and social care services where patients and service users can be identified and would expect that the information will be kept private. This may include, for instance, details about symptoms, diagnosis, treatment, names and addresses. Although the requirement to adhere to these principles is specific to the UK, they are useful across all countries and can support all healthcare professionals in keeping patient information safe.

There are eight principles which can guide health and care professionals. These are regularly reviewed and are available via the office of the National Data Guardian (n.d.) in the UK (www.gov.uk).

Principle 1: Justify the purpose(s) for using confidential information

Principle 2: Use confidential information only when it is necessary

Principle 3: Use the minimum necessary confidential information

Principle 4: Access to confidential information should be on a strict need-to-know basis

Principle 5: Everyone with access to confidential information should be aware of their responsibilities

Principle 6: Comply with the law

Principle 7: The duty to share information for individual care is as important as the duty to protect patient confidentiality

Principle 8: Inform patients and service users about how their confidential information is used

SHARED CARE RECORDS

The increasing use of electronic records has made available additional possibilities for the sharing of information to improve care. Sharing of relevant and proportionate information across healthcare providers is thought to support improved clinical decision making and lead to improved clinical outcomes (O'Hanlon 2017). In addition, they can potentially make a positive impact on population health and in reducing health inequalities through the more efficient use of information to improve access to appropriate services for local populations. In the UK, providers of shared care records work closely with their local populations to ensure that specific local needs are being met. However, there is still some uncertainty regarding whether the sharing of data across systems and organisations (known as interoperability) leads to improved quality of care (Li et al. 2022).

Health and social care professionals must be aware of the shared care records in use in their own location(s) and ensure that they are adequately trained to use them. Clinical colleagues should be actively involved in the development of shared care records, as they are easily able to understand the need to maintain patient confidentiality alongside the benefits of sharing to ensure safety of care.

HOW TO USE AND SHARE INFORMATION WITH CONFIDENCE

Patients and service users have a right to ask how their information is being used and shared. They also have a right to object to the sharing of their information. Organisations must make the principles of this clear, and it is often done via a Privacy Notice on their website. Patients and service users should feel confident that all staff will balance their duty to share relevant and appropriate information alongside their duty to protect individual confidentiality.

If patients or service users object to their information being shared, they should be encouraged to discuss this with their healthcare professionals. All professionals must therefore remain up to date on laws and regulations in this area, as well as be able to confidently explain to patients and service users that in some circumstances, not sharing information could affect the care they receive.

In some circumstances, an individual may not want to share specific pieces of information rather than the whole record. This decision should be respected and recorded. It may also be that an individual is happy for their information to be shared for the purposes of providing direct care, but not for research and planning. It is usually possible for an individual to record this preference, either with the care provider or via national systems.

Sometimes, there is no clear answer about what is relevant or appropriate to share. Professional judgement should be used in such cases, and the decision making clearly recorded. Information Governance and Data Protection specialists (including Caldicott Guardians in UK practice) are often readily available within healthcare organisations to support healthcare professionals with learning and specific questions in this complex area.

FREEDOM OF INFORMATION (FOI) AND SUBJECT ACCESS REQUESTS (SARS)

Most countries will have some legal direction around Freedom of Information. This usually relates to two areas:

- Public authorities being obliged to publish certain information about the work they do
- Members of the public being entitled to request information from public authorities

Having such legislation indicates that a public sector body is open and transparent and increases public trust and confidence. Thus, the default position should be that information is shared when requested. Most public organisations openly provide much of their information via their websites, and it is often possible to gain information via this route, rather than making an official FOI request.

Sometimes, patients and service users mistakenly think that they need to make an FOI request in order to access their own information. However, in the UK, this is actually a data protection subject access request, and it is important that healthcare professionals are able to explain this difference. In other countries, individuals have a right to see their health record and can apply to a healthcare provider to access it. Data protection regulations exist to protect people's right to privacy, whereas FOI legislation is about getting rid of unnecessary secrecy.

In the UK, most healthcare organisations have a department who to support professionals in responding to both FOI and SAR requests, and information about how to contact them will be readily available via their websites and local induction and training.

KEY SUCCESS FACTORS FOR GOOD IG WITHIN AND ACROSS HEALTHCARE ORGANISATIONS

- Organisation-or system-wide strategy – each organisation is different, but there will be common areas when it comes to Information Governance.
- Consistency – across paper and electronic formats.
- Learning and sharing lessons – some organisations will have robust and mature arrangements in place. These should be built upon and used to enhance other areas of a healthcare system.
- Empower colleagues – regular, high-quality training should be provided so that the staff understands their responsibilities.
- Continuous improvement – development and analysis of key performance metrics on information management is key to reaching and exceeding goals.

LEARNING EXERCISE

A person that you have been caring for is concerned that someone in their family has been given access to their medical notes without their permission. What are the formal IG and Data Protection frameworks and processes used to try and ensure that this does not happen?

Cyber Security

Poor data protection and information management can cause personal, social and reputational damage. It is vital that information be available when needed to support care, but it must also be trusted, consistent and accurate so that healthcare professionals can rely on it when providing care.

However, the number of individuals involved in criminal activity is ever increasing. The value of health data is significant and the number of possible entry points to accessing substantial amounts of data makes this a particularly lucrative activity. It is, therefore, vital that all health and care workers are able to keep themselves as safe as possible.

The older technology infrastructure in use in some healthcare organisations makes them especially vulnerable, and this new area of policy and governance is not universally understood; meaning that assurance processes are not always robust. The nature of healthcare services also makes them more vulnerable to criminal attack. In order to provide safe care, the data need to be open and accessible (including records), and this makes them more vulnerable. It is also true that (unlike in other industries) services cannot stop or close when targeted.

There have been several high-profile cyber-attacks in the healthcare sector over recent years, including in the US, the UK, Ireland and Australia. In 2021, hospitals across Ireland lost access to electronic records; services were disrupted, appointments were cancelled, and some medical equipment was disabled. Data had also been compromised. The cybercriminal group claimed it had patient details, employee records and financial information, and reportedly, demanded a ransom of €16.5 m to prevent the release of the data and to decrypt the files (Perlroth et al. 2021). The job of restoring the affected systems was gradual, taking several months for some elements. In 2020, 16% of large UK businesses and charities reported ransomware attacks. This makes responsibilities for cyber security everyone's business.

THREATS TO DATA SECURITY

Social Engineering is where those who want to steal data use tricks or deception to manipulate people into giving access to data. It usually includes a prolonged period of preparation, including reviewing organisational charts and finding employees using popular social media sites. The goal is to gain the trust of one or more employees. All healthcare professionals must be alert for such methods. For example, you should **never** allow colleagues without identification into healthcare facilities and should always check the credentials of phone callers with the office or ward/unit, including when the caller claims that they too work for the organisation. For example, managers and IT departments will **never** ask you to share your login details with them over phone. Also, it is crucial to be mindful of how much information one shares about themselves on social media sites. Ideally, one should **never** share information about their place of work or patients/service users.

E-mail is a highly effective way of transferring information securely, but there are risks in doing so. Criminal hackers sometimes use unsolicited e-mails to try and trick people into disclosing information. If you receive an unsolicited e-mail from an unknown sender, do not open attachments or links you have not requested. E-mails requesting you to input information, including passwords and/or personal and financial details, are highly likely to be an attempt to scam/defraud. Therefore, **never** pass on any information. If you do receive such e-mails, you should report them to your

IT department, who will investigate them. In many organisations, there is a 'Report Phishing' option within the e-mail application for you to do so easily.

GOOD PRACTICE

- Be vigilant when looking at websites. If a web browser says you are about to enter an untrusted site, be very careful. It could be a fake phishing website which has been made to look just like a real one.
- Use strong passwords on all your devices. A good practice is to use different passwords for different sites. You should consider the use of a free password manager. For details on these and other useful information, visit the National Cyber Security Centre (UK) website.
- Be aware of your location. Do not assume that public Wi-Fi networks are secure. Sit where you cannot be overlooked and keep paper documents safe and minimal.
- On your home Wi-Fi network, make sure to change default passwords from those given by your internet provider and consider using encryption, such as WPA2.
- Always disable 'auto connect' to unknown Wi-Fi networks on all your devices.
- Ensure that your devices are up to date with the latest patches and make sure they require a password to unlock them. If you see a device in your work environment which is unlocked, lock it (press the Windows key + L on a Windows PC/laptop). Remind your colleagues about the risks of leaving devices unlocked, especially if they are used for confidential patient information.

The layers of security we rely on in the workplace reduce when working remotely. Threat actors (criminals engaged in cyber-crime) are well aware that people are increasingly working remotely, which presents an opportunity for them to exploit. All of the information above is just as useful in both personal and professional life, irrespective of your physical location.

CYBER SECURITY AND CONNECTED MEDICAL DEVICES

Due to the risks involved in patient safety, medical devices are highly regulated and controlled. Modifications, including to software and hardware, need to be authorised by the medical device manufacturer, who will have conducted extensive validation and verification procedures in line with the regulations. Therefore, using medical devices on clinical networks has some specific cyber security issues, including difficulties in upgrading operating systems, greater software complexity (employing multiple means of connectivity) and a greater pressure to keep the device available. There can also be issues related to the length of time it takes for security patches to become available. There is significant potential for criminals to exploit all these factors. Security incidents affecting connected medical devices can cause significant disruption to the delivery of healthcare services.

All healthcare organisations must be alert for these additional risks and enact mitigations, including not allowing use of medical devices for end-user activities (such as email or web browsing). Organisations need to consider and constrain data flows to medical servers wherever possible and ensure that multi-factor authentication (MFA) is used by any supplier remotely connecting to their network (NHS Digital 2022).

The impact of any cyber incident in this area is significant and all healthcare organisations must have suitable Business Continuity Processes (BCP) and Disaster Recovery (DR) plans in place. Healthcare professionals should familiarise themselves with these processes and ensure that staff training includes sufficient information about how to stay protected.

LEARNING EXERCISE

Imagine a criminal gang has successfully compromised your digital systems, and there has been a complete shutdown of your digital patient records. You are unable to use any of your medical devices. Identify your organisation's BCP and DR plans and consider what strategies you would need to put in place to ensure you can continue to deliver safe patient care while the systems are out of action.

CASE STUDY

Nursing staff in a hospice did not have access to the recent medical history of their new patients. Each time a new patient was admitted, the hospice needed to telephone their primary care provider (GP practice) to request information about their recent care. One or more clinical teams in the local hospital were often also caring for the patients and requesting information about the patient via telephone or e-mail. This resulted in delays in providing care, and on some occasions, impacting patient safety, since timely access to nursing observations and medicines/allergy information was needed urgently on admission.

To make the process more efficient, the local care system (including the hospice) agreed to a collaborative data sharing agreement, so that nursing and other clinical staff would have access to their patients' electronic medical records, when necessary. All the different providers across the Integrated Care System (ICS) made patients aware that if their care was being provided across this system, then there was a possibility that clinicians working in different organisations would access their clinical records. In addition, on admission, the patients' explicit consent, or that of their representatives, was requested before their record was accessed. Where consent to access electronic records was not provided, the former system of contacting the primary care provider or hospital would continue to be used.

Other key features of the data sharing agreement were:
- access to records could only take place while they were under the care of the hospice;
- access was restricted to the clinical and professional nursing staff at the hospice;
- access was only allowed when this was necessary to provide treatment and for patients' safety;
- access was restricted to information relevant to the provision of care;
- access to the information was by secure means; and
- the information obtained was held securely and in accordance with good information management practice.

Conclusion

This chapter identified the key principles of IG and cyber security that nurses need to consider when caring for people in a digital environment. It highlighted the importance of the frameworks that are put in place to ensure that data about care is safe, and only shared with individuals who need to access that data. It also highlighted the importance of providing information to people about how their data are being used and shared and ensuring where appropriate that their consent is obtained before sharing.

Nurses also need to be aware of the issues surrounding cyber security. The risks to organisations and data are increasing, with the increasing use of digital technologies in healthcare settings. Ensuring they are aware of the potential risks associated with their use of digital technology, and being vigilant when using and communicating via digital means are important for keeping information safe.

Key Points

1. Health and social care professionals have a legal and professional duty to share information to support individual care.
2. They must share only relevant and necessary information and check for a person's objections and transfer information securely.
3. They professionals must utilise skilled individuals within local, regional and national organisations to support decision making where appropriate.
4. They must maintain the same standards across all areas of personal and professional life.
5. They must maintain up-to-date practice. The risks and mitigations change often. Health and social care professionals must attend regular training to maintain safe practice.

References

NHS Digital, 2022. Guidance on Protecting Connected Medical Devices. Available at: https://digital.nhs.uk/cyber-and-data-security/guidance-and-assurance/guidance-on-protecting-connected-medical-devices.

Ham, C., Charles, A., Wellings, D., 2018. Shared Responsibility for Health: The Cultural Change We Need. The King's Fund. Available at: https://www.kingsfund.org.uk/publications/shared-responsibility-health.

Li, E., Clarke, J., Ashrafian, H., et al., 2022. The impact of electronic health record interoperability on safety and quality of care in high-income countries: systematic review. J. Med. Internet Res. 24 (9), e38144. https://doi.org/10.2196/38144.

National Data Guardian, n.d. The Caldicott principles. Available at: https://www.gov.uk/government/publications/the-caldicott-principles.

O'Hanlon, S., 2017. Why Data Sharing Matters For Excellent Care. NHS Confederation. Available at: https://www.nhsconfed.org/articles/why-data-sharing-matters-excellent-care.

Perlroth, N., Satariano, A., 2021. Irish Hospitals Are Latest to Be Hit By Ransomware Attacks. The New York Times. Available at: https://www.nytimes.com/2021/05/20/techn ology/ransomware-attack-ireland-hospitals.html.

Royal College of Nursing, 2022. Available at: https://www.rcn.org.uk/clinical-topics/eHealth/Information-governance.

Recommendations for Further Reading

General Data Protection Regulations, n.d. GDPR. Available at: https://gdpr-info.eu/.

Health Information Portability and Accountability Act of 1996, n.d. HIPAA Home. Available at: hhs.gov.

National Cyber Security Centre, n.d. About cyber essentials. Available at: https://www.ncsc .gov.uk/cyberessentials/overview.

NHS Digital, n.d. Cyber and data security awareness and resources. Available at: https://digital.nhs.uk/cyber-and-data-security/services?area=guidance-and-assurance.

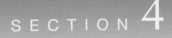

SECTION 4

Advancing Practice through Digitally Enabled Innovation and Research

SECTION OUTLINE

CHAPTER 12

Harnessing Improvement Science for Digitally Enabled Nursing and Midwifery

Gillian Janes ■ Lisa Ward

At the end of the chapter, the nurses will be able to:

- Demonstrate a critical understanding of the role of improvement science in enabling health improvement using digital solutions.
- Explore how nurses and midwives can use improvement science within the context of digitally enabled quality improvement and their own contribution to this agenda.
- Apply an improvement methodology to effectively support quality improvement in their own digital practice context.

Introduction

This chapter explores the concept of improvement science and its relevance for nurses and midwives seeking to reap the benefits of digital solutions to improve healthcare services. It considers possible applications of a quality improvement (QI) approach, illustrated using a case study. The case study takes the example of introducing e-observations in an adult in-patient care setting. However, the improvement principles applied in the development of this new way of working are equally applicable to other digitally enabled improvements and clinical contexts. This chapter will enable nurses and midwives to consider their own QI expertise, including their approach to leading change, by providing guided learning activities that will enable them to examine how these transferable knowledge and skills can be applied to support improved services and health outcomes within the context of their own digital health practice.

IMPROVEMENT SCIENCE AND ITS RELEVANCE FOR DIGITALLY ENABLED PRACTICE

Nurses and midwives must not only practise safely and effectively (NMC 2018) but also be able to work with people, carers and colleagues to improve work processes and ultimately, population health outcomes. Following the recognition of QI as an integral part of modern healthcare, recent decades have seen a focus on the development

117

of QI capacity in the workforce (Dixon-Woods 2019). More recently, a substantial potential of developing and applying appropriate digital solutions to enhance the quality and resilience of healthcare services, population health and wellbeing, has been recognised internationally (WHO 2022). Capitalising on this potential is now a priority to address the challenges associated with meeting increasing and complex population health needs and shifting public expectations.

Improvement science can be defined as:

> *...exploring how to undertake quality improvement well. It inhabits the sphere between research and quality improvement by applying research methods to help understand what impacts on quality improvement.*

(The Health Foundation 2011:3)

Facilitating improvement is a complex, non-linear process that requires the integrated application of a range of theories and practical tools alongside transferable nursing knowledge and skills (Janes et al. 2022). This is the case for any improvement effort and the principles are the same, irrespective of whether the improvement involves a digital component. For example, improvement science can be used to:

- guide the design and commissioning of digital solutions to ensure optimal care processes and usability (i.e. to avoid digitising poor processes or work design).
- support optimisation of digital solutions following initial large-scale implementation, which would traditionally use a change methodology, such as PRINCE 2.

Improvement methodologies are designed to guide a systematic approach to change, which is particularly important within complex settings such as healthcare. Though a range of alternative methodologies are available, there is no evidence that one is necessarily better than another (Alderwick et al. 2017). This chapter focuses on applying The Model for Improvement (MFI) (Langley et al. 2009) for illustration purposes. The hugely influential Institute for Healthcare Improvement defines improvement science as:

> *... an applied science that emphasises innovation, rapid cycle testing in the field and spread...to generate learning about what changes, in what contexts produce improvements. It is characterized by the combination of expert subject knowledge with improvement methods and tools. It is multidisciplinary, drawing on clinical science, systems theory, psychology, statistics and other fields.*

(IHI 2022)

Reflecting this definition, the MFI (Langley et al. 2009) has become synonymous with Improvement Science and is used internationally to promote sustainable, continuous improvement. This model was designed to support data-driven, small-scale, emergent and sustainable change using rapid-cycle testing, learning and re-testing in the field. This enables proximal knowledge generation by and for local health populations and issues (Clarke et al. 2002), which makes it particularly relevant for guiding practitioner-led improvement. One advantage of the MFI is that evaluation is embedded throughout, with data generated during implementation and used to guide subsequent cycles. This reduces risk and potential waste of resources on promising but non-viable change ideas. Used appropriately, therefore, the MFI offers a rigorous, experimental approach to improvement, addressing complex problems and responding to the unforeseen impact of change (Reed et al. 2016).

Despite being widely and successfully used in healthcare, the simplicity of the MFI, which is highly attractive, belies the complexity involved. This can hinder effective application in practice, particularly by those new to QI. A new, explanatory version of the MFI, offered by Janes et al. (2022) to provide a more detailed illustration to support its practical application, is therefore used here to illustrate the application of the MFI in case study (see Fig. 12.1).

The MFI (Langley et al. 2009) is a structured two-part framework. Part one comprises three questions:

What are we trying to accomplish?

How will we know that change represents an improvement?

What changes can we make that will lead to improvement?

Responding to the questions in part one of the MFI lays the foundations for part two by prompting the identification of a specific improvement aim (question 1), evaluation criteria and measures (question 2) and finally, the change to be tested (question 3).

Part two of the model, the **P**lan **D**o **C**heck **A**dapt/Abandon/Adopt (**PDCA**) cycle, concerns implementation. Here, changes designed to achieve improvement are planned, implemented, tested, iterated and then gradually scaled up using multiple cycles, based on the learning from the Check (evaluation) phase of each cycle. How the cycles are best iterated is specific to a particular improvement. For example, the first PDCA cycle could involve just one person's care process or experience, with subsequent cycles involving adjusting the actual intervention, increasing the number of people involved (patients and/or staff) and/or testing in different environments until all stakeholders are satisfied that no further refinements are necessary, or that the idea should be abandoned.

APPLYING IMPROVEMENT SCIENCE IN DIGITAL NURSING PRACTICE

The following case study and Fig. 12.1 illustrate how the MFI (Langley et al. 2009) was used in practice to enable digital transformation. This example demonstrates that used appropriately, the MFI offers a rigorous, experimental approach to improvement, allowing complex improvement problems to be tackled whilst simultaneously addressing the identification and management of any unforeseen impact (Reed et al. 2016). This ensures that patient safety is maintained throughout the process and is ultimately enhanced because of the change. The iterative, cyclical testing and evaluation is also more likely to achieve buy-in or support from colleagues who might otherwise be suspicious or unsupportive of change.

Q1: What are we trying to accomplish? **To improve the early recognition of patient deterioration and reduce avoidable cardiac arrests and deaths.**

Q2: How will We know that a change is an improvement? **There will be increased accuracy of NEWS calculation and adherence to escalation policy, sustained reduction in cardiac arrests and reduction in instances of failure to rescue.**

Q3: What change can we make that will result in improvement? **Implement an electronic observation platform to facilitate recognition of patient deterioration and support early escalation**

ADOPT: Integrate into routine operations and organisational surveillance processes

Cycle 1: Pilot implementation e-obs and NEWS2	
P	Identify two pilot wards. Brief staff and prepare for change.
D	Commence the pilot under close monitoring
C	Emergency calls, staff feedback and patient data analysis demonstrate over alerting causing problems for clinical staff and may compromise patient safety.
A	Pause pilot. Revert to EWS matrix and paper observation charts. Develop revised plan

Cycle 2: Second Pilot implementation e-obs and EWS	
P	Work with the supplier to embed the existing EWS matrix into the digital platform and provide pilot ward staff with additional training
D	Commence the pilot (revised scoring tool) underclose monitoring
C	Emergency calls, staff feedback and patient data analysis indicate the pilot is adding benefit for staff and patient safety is maintained.
A	Roll out to full organisational implementation

Cycle 3: Organisation wide roll out e-obs and EWS parameter testing	
P	Develop and agree roll-out plan for full organisational implementation, including compilation of information it an understandable format to enable decision making with ongoing monitoring of impact.
D	Complete roll-out implementation with ongoing patient data monitoring, staff feedback analysis and comparison of possible escalation parameters
C	Data analysis indicates appropriate escalation, no patient safety risk and positive staff benefits.
A	Present the information to multiple stakeholder groups, obtain expert advice and agree to build the NEWS2 matrix and chosen escalation points into the digital platform.

Cycle 4: Transition to NEWS2	
P	Work with the supplier to build the NEWS2 matrix and chosen escalation points into the digital platform. All clinical areas educated on the NEWS2 scoring matrix and escalation parameters. Extensive communications/engagement campaign.
D	Switch over from EWS to NEWS2 on a defined date and time. Continue collection and analysis of emergency calls, staff feedback and patient data.
C	Data indicates that the pilot is adding benefit and patient safety is maintained
A	Move to routine operation and review through ongoing audit.

Key: P = plan, D = do, C = check, A = act/adapt/abandon

Fig. 12.1 Application of The Model for Improvement, explanatory version (Adapted from Janes et al. 2022)

CASE STUDY

Nurse-led quality improvement: Evolution from paper-based to electronic physiological observations recording and automated escalation using a mobile digital solution.

The improvement took place in, and was led by senior nurses at, a large integrated Trust. Significant work had already been completed using The Model for Improvement (Langley et al. 2009) to enhance the detection and management of deteriorating patients and reduce the number of cardiac arrests. The subsequent introduction of electronic observations and escalation resulted in a 14% drop in cardiac arrests, the biggest single in-year reduction of a total 46% reduction/1000 admissions over a seven-year period. The move to an e-observation platform incorporated a planned transition from using the locally developed Early Warning Scoring (EWS) matrix to the National Early Warning Score (NEWS2); this was perceived as the most seamless and effective way to support the change to the new aggregate scoring tool.

The key benefit of electronic observations is removing potential human error in calculating and aggregating NEWS, taking accuracy to 100% (Lockwood et al. 2020) and reducing the risk of unrecognised patient deterioration. Prior to large-scale implementation, the new system was piloted on two respiratory wards. This indicated, however, that patients were repeatedly alerting for escalation, which resulted in significant numbers on very high-frequency observations and staff struggling to differentiate alerts from real patient deterioration. Investigation of a near miss incident identified that with the old EWS matrix, the patient would have triggered an emergency call on four occasions over a 24-hour period. However, using NEWS2 in the e-observation system, the same patient would NOT have triggered an emergency call on four occasions. This raised significant concerns for patient safety due to emerging evidence of alert fatigue. The pilot was therefore paused, and the staff reverted to using the original EWS matrix. This enabled continued safe implementation and scale-up of e-observations and easy capture of this data, which was then used to explore how NEWS2 could be safely implemented.

Following Trust-wide rollout of the e-observation platform, data analysis and benchmarking against the Welsh Rapid Response to Acute Illness (RRAILS) Programme was used to determine the most appropriate escalation triggers to support the management of deteriorating patients most effectively. This analysis indicated that using the low (3), medium (6) and high (9) risk escalation scores implemented as part of the RRAILS programme (Hancock 2015), rather than RCP (2017) recommended escalation at scores of 5 and 7, would be safe and effective. NEWS2 was therefore implemented using RRAILS-based escalation criteria over four years ago and on-going audit of deteriorating patients and cardiac arrests since then ensures constant surveillance, which continues to indicate these escalation points remain appropriate. Figure 12.1 illustrates this improvement process.

APPLYING QI SKILLS IN DIGITAL NURSING PRACTICE

This case study illustrates some key principles in the application of QI methodology for digital transformation by nurses in the clinical environment, though these are not specific to digital improvement. This section explores some of these within the three foundational aspects, or pillars, of improvement outlined in the conceptual model of QI proposed by Janes et al. (2022): context, core skills and tools and strategies.

Consider the Context

The organisation and teams involved in the case study had previously experienced improvement work in the organisation, using the same improvement methodology, that is, the MFI. This familiarity with the methodology and positive change experience had enabled the staff leading this change to develop trusting, well-established relationships with the staff and stakeholders involved. This provided a sure foundation for the change process and enabled the high level of staff engagement and open communication required for success. For example, one of the nurses leads discovered the problem with over-alerting associated with the PDCA cycle 1 change during an informal conversation with a very junior member of staff working on one of the pilot wards. This illustrates the benefits of nursing and midwifery leaders making themselves available and being genuinely accepting of critical feedback, which can help staff feel psychologically safe and confident enough to raise genuine concerns (RCN 2021).

Use Core Skills

Core improvement skills are in two main categories: technical improvement skills and personal leadership skills. Whilst technical knowledge of improvement is important, regardless of the improvement methodology used, the leadership skills employed in its application in practice are often the difference between success and failure. Even with a relatively straightforward methodology like the MFI, and though not explicit in the case study description, the skills of the clinicians leading the improvement described are crucial. These reflect the compassionate, inclusive and collective leadership that is known to be central to high-quality care and enabling the supportive culture required to achieve this (Oxlade 2020). The importance of developing an improvement culture that includes creating psychological safety as central to this is illustrated in the example above.

Even in the case study described, however, where there was previous positive experience of change and use of the MFI methodology, it was important to start small, by piloting the incorporation of NEWS2 into the new electronic system on two wards to begin with. This enabled the early identification of the unforeseen impact on patient safety and staff wellbeing and provides a good example of why starting small, even in a change-positive environment or with what seems like an obvious improvement idea, is crucial. This is particularly important in the context of the current NHS with a fatigued and depleted workforce, compounded by increasingly complex health needs and unprecedented demand for services. As the case study clearly illustrates, this approach can provide early indications of increased patient safety risks and enable the improvement plan to be paused to allow for adaptation and testing of alternative solutions, whilst maintaining service delivery.

Despite the increasing use of automation and digitisation, healthcare remains a predominantly human-centric endeavour, often involving highly complex work processes. Progress is being made in recognising the importance of designing healthcare work systems and equipment that account for the intrinsic fallibility of humans to reduce errors and support staff wellbeing.

Concerned with the dynamic interaction between the task and environment in which it takes place, the discipline of Human Factors (or Ergonomics) is defined as the development of:

...rigorous, elegant, evidence-based solutions to problems and building resilient systems that enable people to do the right things, every time.

(CIEHF 2019:2)

This includes, for example, applying design and behavioural science to the design of equipment and work processes, including individual human characteristics and interaction with other members of the team. The aim is to make it easy to do the right thing; therefore, applying Human Factors/Ergonomics to the design and implementation of any potential solution is crucial, not least for any improvement involving digital or technological change.

Starting small can also enable leaders to develop the shared vision and stakeholder commitment or buy-in needed to effect any sustainable change. In a complex environment like healthcare, where improvement often aims to address 'wicked problems', effective leaders need to engage, understand what motivates and influence others. Goyder (2014) introduces the concept of 'Gravitas' as key to enabling individuals to lead with confidence, command trust and respect, and inspire others:

Gravitas = Knowledge + Purpose + Passion − Anxiety

Knowledge, purpose and passion are plentiful in nursing and midwifery; however, so too is anxiety, with all four fluctuating in response to a range of factors. This means nurses and midwives are not always good at maximising their contribution to improvement work or recognising how this enhances healthcare outcomes. Framing how they think about their expertise and contribution to improvement using the Gravitas equation can help to overcome the 'imposter syndrome' that many nurses and midwives feel; this would enable them to exert their improvement leadership ability regardless of their role, thereby supporting the leadership at every level for the delivery of consistent, high-quality services. Completing the learning activities at the end of this chapter will enable you to undertake a self-assessment of your expertise in these areas and develop a development plan to enhance these.

Use Appropriate Tools and Strategies

Information on a wide range of improvement tools and strategies is plentiful and easily accessible (see, for example: https://www.england.nhs.uk/sustainableimprovement/qsir-programme/qsir-tools/). Data, however, is an important improvement tool that is often overlooked but must be effectively used alongside other, perhaps more readily known tools, like process mapping or stakeholder analysis. Data provides relevant means of:

- identifying good practice to spread or a problem to be addressed
- evaluating progress during an improvement and guiding further adjustments to the process, including the identification of unintended consequences (positive and negative)

• monitoring effectiveness once an improvement is established.

Whilst nurses and midwives are exceptionally good at telling the story of the need for change or the change process itself, they can lack confidence in where to obtain and how to use data, often holding to the misconception that it is not relevant to their work. A key part of leading any quality improvement is engaging the teams involved in understanding the power of data and how it can be employed to improve care. As described in the case study, data was used for two main purposes: to ensure patient safety is maintained throughout and help determine the final solution. This case study reinforces the importance of improvement leaders keeping an open mind regarding the actual change required and end point of any digitally based QI. Furthermore, it illustrates that data collected during one improvement can be used to support another. Based on the adage 'Data makes us credible, stories make us memorable', the quantitative data and patient stories collected during the ongoing evaluation of the change described in the case study were combined and used by one of the clinical leads to build a successful business case for a new, bespoke service to support deteriorating and dying patients. This enabled further improvements to the service and had the additional benefit of supporting the development of an improvement culture as the routine use of data to enhance service delivery and outcomes becomes part of everyday clinical practice.

LEARNING EXERCISES

1. Reflect on how this chapter has reinforced or enhanced your previous QI knowledge and experience, and identify three actions you could take to apply this learning within the context of your role; for example, contact a QI specialist in your organisation.
2. Review the nine domains of the Healthcare Leadership Model at http s://www.leadershipacademy.nhs.uk/resources/healthcare-leadership-model/supporting-tools-resources/healthcare-leadership-model-self-assessment-tool/ and complete the self-assessment questionnaire (if you have already done so in the last six months, use that). Based on either the case study above or your own experience of leading improvement in a digital context, consider:
   • Which of the nine domains is your strength? How might you use this more effectively to lead the digital agenda?
   • Which of the nine domains would you like to enhance your knowledge and skills in? What three actions could you take to support your further development in this area?

Conclusion

This chapter has explored the concept of improvement science and its relevance for nurses and midwives seeking to improve healthcare services by using digital solutions. It has also outlined possible applications of a QI approach within the context of digital transformation. An example of improving care quality using digital solutions has been used to illustrate how an internationally recognised and commonly used improvement methodology, the MFI (Langley et al. 2009) was used to facilitate improvement, including the safe and effective management of unintended consequences of change. Regardless of the improvement methodology used, however, nursing and midwifery leadership is crucial in the context of its application. Some key considerations in this regard have been discussed within the context of the case study and the learning activities contained in the chapter provide nurses and midwives the opportunity to examine and develop a plan for how to enhance their own improvement leadership expertise, whilst capitalising on their transferable knowledge and skills. Digital transformation offers great potential for enhancing patient, staff and organisational outcomes and experiences. However, any potential gains are only likely to be achieved if nurses and midwives develop their improvement science expertise and use their transferable leadership skills in its application.

Key Points

1. Quality improvement is a core part of every nursing and midwifery role.
2. Improvement Science is highly relevant for enabling healthcare services improvement that involves digital solutions.
3. The Model for Improvement can be appropriately applied and highly effective when used to support change in a range of digital transformation contexts.
4. Stakeholder involvement and the application of Human Factors science/Ergonomics in the design and implementation of digital solutions is crucial to ensure effectiveness and the usability necessary to sustain the change in the longer term.
5. Nurses and midwives have transferable leadership, change management and clinical expertise that are critical for supporting effective digital transformation.

References

Alderwick, H., Charles, A., Jones, B., et al., 2017. Making the Case for Quality Improvement: Lessons for NHS Boards and Leaders. The King's Fund, London.
CIEHF, 2019. Human Factors and Healthcare Evidencing the Impact of Human Factors Training to Support Improvements in Patient Safety and to Contribute to Cultural Change. Chartered Institute of Ergonomics and Human Factors, Wootton Wawen.
Clarke, C.L., Wilcockson, J., 2002. Seeing need and developing care: exploring knowledge for and from practice. Int. J. Nurs. Stud. 39, 397–406.
Dixon-Woods, M., 2019. How to improve healthcare improvement: an essay by Mary Dixon-Woods. BMJ. 366, l5514. https://doi.org/10.1136/bmj.l5514.
Goyder, C., 2014. Gravitas: Communicate with Confidence, Influence and Authority. Vermilion, London.
Hancock, C., 2015. A national quality improvement initiative for reducing harm and death from sepsis in Wales. Intensive Crit. Care Nurs. 31 (2), 100–105. https://doi.org/10.1016/j.iccn.2014.11.004.

IHI, 2022. Science of Improvement. Institute for Healthcare Improvement. Available at: htt ps://www.ihi.org/about/Pages/ScienceofImprovement.aspx#:~:text=The%20science%20o f%20improvement%20is,with%20improvement%20methods%20and%20tools.

Janes, G., Delves-Yates, C., 2022. Foundations chapter. In: Janes, G., Delves-Yates, C. (Eds.), Quality Improvement in Nursing. Sage, London.

Langley, G.L., Moen, R., Nolan, T.W., et al., 2009. The Improvement Guide: A Practical Approach to Enhancing Organizational Performance, second ed. Jossey-Bass, San-Francisco.

Lockwood, M., Thomas, J., Martin, S., et al., 2020. AutoPEWS: automating pediatric early warning score calculation improves accuracy without sacrificing predictive ability. Pediatr. Qual. Saf. 5 (2), e274. https://doi.org/10.1097/pq9.0000000000000274.

NMC, 2018. The Code: Professional Standards of Practice and Behaviour for Nurses, Midwives and Nursing Associates. Nursing and Midwifery Council, London.

Oxlade, L., 2020. The Courage of Compassion: Supporting Nurses and Midwives to Deliver High-Quality Care. The King's Fund, London.

RCN, 2021. Nursing Workforce Standards: Supporting a Safe and Effective Nursing Workforce. Royal College of Nursing, London.

RCP, 2017. National Early Warning Score (NEWS) 2: Standardising the Assessment of Acute-Illness Severity in the NHS. Royal College of Physicians, London. https://www.rcplondon.ac.uk/projects/outputs/national-early-warning-score-news-2

Reed, J.E., Card, A.J., 2016. The problem with plan-do-study-act cycles. BMJ Qual. Saf. 25 (3), 147–152. https://doi.org/10.1136/bmjqs-2015-005076.

The Health Foundation, 2011. Evidence Scan: Improvement Science. The Health Foundation, London.

WHO, 2022. Regional Digital Health Action Plan for the WHO European Region 2023–2030. World Health Organization. Regional Office for Europe, Geneva.

CHAPTER 13

Using Data to Drive Improvement

Helen Balsdon

LEARNING OUTCOMES

At the end of this chapter, the nurses will be able to:
- Understand how nursing and midwifery leaders use data.
- Consider the different types of data required for local improvement projects.
- Describe how data is evolving and the implications for practice.
- Understand what data quality is and the qualities of good data.

Introduction

In an increasingly digital era, change is a certainty. Nurses generate the largest amount of data of any healthcare professional (Collins et al. 2018). It is thus essential that this data be used to change practice for patient benefit and to continually evolve as a profession.

Using data for improvement may appear a modern nursing concept, but it is not. Nurses have a longstanding culture of using data for improvement. In the mid-19th century, one of Florence Nightingale's many achievements included collecting and analysing data, presenting it in a way that could be easily interpreted and using it to influence change (Stacey and Westwood 2022).

Digital maturity of health and care services around the world is rapidly increasing, accelerated by the Covid pandemic. This brings nursing and midwifery to an inflection point, where they need to learn to incorporate digitally generated data into everyday practice and use it to improve care. However, sources of data are also evolving. Although there is growing awareness that digital technologies will enable and support improvements to care, there is also uncertainty about how this can be harnessed safely and effectively.

This chapter explores how leaders use data, explores data quality and discusses the role nurses and midwives have in this. It also considers how digital technology will evolve data and discusses the implication for clinical practice.

HOW NURSE AND MIDWIFE LEADERS USE DATA

Information needs of nursing and midwifery leaders are wide and varied. The purpose of data and its use may differ at the different layers of an organisation, from the point of care to the boardroom.

Generally, the purposes of data for nursing and midwifery leaders falls into four key areas:

- Quality and safety
- Performance and compliance
- Improvements or change initiatives
- Organisational change or service reconfiguration

Data may serve internal requirements whilst also seeking to provide assurance to external stakeholders, such as regulators. This is not always mutually exclusive. For example, leaders will want to understand the safety of the services. Some of this information may also be provided to the regulator for external assurance. Table 13.1 gives some examples of data that may be used for different purposes.

Commonly, multiple types of data are collated and presented to show the trend over time. This may require business intelligence tools to extract data from multiple sources and present it for easy interpretation. For example, a chief nurse may want to know how many falls there were, how many resulted in harm, and of what level (minor to catastrophic). This type of information is usually presented in a table containing monthly data for a rolling 12 months, making it possible to identify trends over time. The next layer of data for falls may be by location. Quantitative data may also be accompanied by explanatory notes to contextualize the situation, explain variation or outline the actions taken.

Data are becoming a core part of healthcare and used by nurses and midwives in daily practice. Despite this, the current way in which nurses and midwives access data is not without challenges. For example, manual data collection can be time consuming, leaving little time for the professionals to consider what the data is showing or for using it to inform improvements. Additionally, as digital data is not always easy to access, this can be a barrier. Accessing digital data often requires requests to information technology services and can involve drawing data from multiple digital systems. Digital tools are required to do this extraction efficiently and to present the information in a way that aids interpretation.

Data quality can also be a challenge. Data quality is defined as data being good enough to support the outcomes it is being used for (Government Data Hub 2021). Qualities of good data are completeness, uniqueness, consistency, timeliness, validity, accuracy (Government Data Hub 2021). Key considerations in assessing data quality include understanding the definitions and assumptions, so that the data mean the same thing to all who use it. Assuring good data quality starts when data is entered into a system at the point of care. For example, using a structured tool to record vital signs or an assessment, so that the data is recorded in the same way each time, regardless of who records the information. However, it is not always possible to record all the care in a structured format. Instead, narrative may be more appropriate. Interpreting narrative or observational data often requires an element of professional judgement. In these cases, the data quality may vary, as each person may consider a situation differently. This does not mean these types of data should not be used. However, as advocated by the Institute of Healthcare Improvement (IHI) model of improvement,

TABLE 13.1 ■ **Data Used by Nurse and Midwife Leaders**

Purpose	Type of Data	Examples	Potential Source of Data
Quality and safety	Quantitative	Incidence of different types of infections by type; Number of falls with harm	Electronic health record (EHR), risk management data system
Performance and compliance	Quantitative	Number of inpatient admissions to a hospital; Percentage of complaints responded to within a defined time period	Hospital administration system, EHR, patient experience database
Improvement project	Quantitative and/or qualitative	Improving care, experience, efficiency and productivity. Examples include: Reducing falls on a ward; Improving experience of care on a ward; Improving stock management; Reducing time between decision to discharge and actual discharge time	Local data collection, observations of practice, written feedback, risk management system, EPR
Organisational change	Quantitative and/or qualitative	Number of people using service past, present and anticipated future demand, clinical pathways, financial data	Human resource records, service level data, business cases, finance

it may be prudent to use both qualitative and quantitative data to minimise bias or potential variation (Langley et al. 2009).

There is often a perception in nursing and midwifery that data collected about care will be used to judge or manage performance, as opposed to creating insights or being used for improvement. It is hard to know where this comes from, but for transparency, it is important that the purpose, definitions and data use are clear. This is especially important when using the same datasets for multiple purposes.

USING DATA FOR IMPROVEMENT

Shah (2019) wrote about how best to use data for improvement and stressed that this should be based on the question that the improvement project seeks to answer.

He suggested that when using data for improvement, rarely will one size fit all. In practical terms, a project will often include initial scoping to determine what is already known and what is already collected. The key question then is, will this help answer the question? It is important that the methodology chosen for each improvement project reflects the purpose. There are many purposes that data may be needed for, including local improvement projects, audits, service evaluation and research.

The IHI model for improvement recognises that both qualitative and quantitative data are critical to evaluating and guiding improvement (Langley et al. 2009). The model advocates the use of a range of metrics for a rounded perspective, including outcome, process, and balancing metrics. Outcome metrics measure the performance of what is in study. Process metrics measure whether an activity has happened. Balancing metrics help identify unintended consequences. More about the model for improvement can be found in the chapter Chapter 12.

THE EVOLUTION OF DATA AND THE IMPLICATIONS FOR PRACTICE

Data is evolving with increased digitisation, which is leading to a vast range of technical developments. Alongside this, there is a changing demand for data and information. There is increased focus on population health, and data will be key to driving system-level change to health and care services. Together, all these changes will build reliance on data-driven insights to inform service planning and decision making across healthcare systems. It is therefore important for nurses and midwives to understand these and how they may impact practice. Evolutions in data we expect to see include:

Standards and Interoperability

People have multiple interactions with health and care providers in a range of locations. The professionals will each make a written record of the interaction. As the electronic health record (EHR) in use in each location varies, the records of one individual will be in many different systems. Additionally, the language and abbreviations used may be different in each location. Abbreviations may have a different meaning in different care settings or in different parts of the world. This happens because of varying working contexts.

Information standards can help address this issue, as they can support in reducing unwarranted variation. Information standards support a consistent way of recording, define the structure of the data, type of information to be recorded and the clinical terminology that underpins this. Additionally, the technical specification supports the movement of the message between different EHRs so that it can be easily interpreted and means the same thing to all professionals, wherever the location (NHS Digital 2022).

According to The King's Fund research, there is no universally accepted definition of interoperability (The King's Fund 2022). However, according to the NHS England Interoperability handbook (NHS England 2015), interoperability is the technical term used to describe the movement of information between two systems, in a way that is understandable by both.

Together, standards and interoperability can support a reduction in documentation burden. They define what needs to be recorded (standards) and support the movement of information between care settings in a way that can be understood (interoperability). For nurses and midwives, sharing information digitally makes it possible to work smarter as a collective. It enables building on what has been recorded by others, rather than starting all over again. An example of this would be when a person living in a nursing home attends a hospital. If information about their functional needs and care requirements are moved digitally, using agreed standards and interoperability, this information can be used as the basis of an assessment, rather than having to complete a new assessment. The caveat here is that having the data does not negate the need to use professional judgement to determine if it is appropriate to use. For example, there is a big difference between using data last updated a few days ago versus that recorded years ago.

There are a few dependencies with using standards and interoperability. This includes the requirement for nurses and midwives to use structured rather than narrative data. Structured data can be more easily found and moved digitally between EHRs. For many, this is a big cultural shift as they have used traditionally written narratives to explain their work. There is also a need for nurses and midwives to trust each other's documentation. The King's Fund (2022) research found that making interoperability work effectively was not only about technology but also relationships and an enabling environment. This issue of trust and collaborative working between organisations was also identified as an enabling factor for interoperability in this research (The King's Fund 2022). This clearly articulates the need to align people, process and technology, which are the cornerstones of digital transformation.

The way in which data is generated accounts for many of the changes we can expect to see in a digital future. Changes include medical device integration, predictive (or advanced) analytics, machine learning and artificial intelligence (AI), voice recognition, ambient monitoring and patient entered data.

Medical Device Integration

Medical device integration (MDI) is a software that automatically collects data from different machines and integrates it into the EHR. This allows for a smooth flow of large volumes of data across systems. This is commonly seen within critical care and theatre facilities where there are multiple technologies being used to monitor a person's physical condition. From a nursing and midwifery perspective, having data generated this way removes the need to repeatedly record data manually. However, there remains a need to validate the data to confirm its accuracy. This is a change to the way nurses or midwives work and another area where trust is required, in both the data and the process. However, this is straightforward to achieve, as the machines are all close by, to check the machinery, confirm what the EHR shows and make comparisons. This technology has the potential to release time to care, allowing the nurses or midwives to focus on other aspects of care that are required.

Predictive (or Advanced) Analytics

Predictive analytics involves the use of data to predict future trends, events or risks. This is a software that uses an algorithm to search digital systems, in most cases the EHR, for pre-identified data relevant to different scenarios. Examples of use in nursing include using EHR data to predict those who may be at risk of acute deterioration or falls. Typically, such tools look at a wide range of data, much more than a traditional assessment tool may include, and present this for clinical review. Predictive analytics can help save nurses/midwives time and reduce documentation burden. However, it is important to ensure that the algorithm has a robust evidence base and looks at all the relevant data. It is also important that the information is presented in a way that helps see where the technology thinks there is a risk, that is, it is explicit about all factors considered, rather than just informing the nurse/midwife that a person is at risk. Using predictive analytics should guide professional decision making about the relative risk and the required actions needed. However, the computer is not always right, and it is important to look at the physical person, and not rely on data alone.

Machine Learning and Artificial Intelligence (AI)

AI is defined as 'the science and engineering of making intelligent machines, especially intelligent computer programs' (McCarthy 1956). Many of us will unknowingly encounter AI when we use the internet. Within healthcare, machine learning and AI are increasingly being adopted to improve efficiency, especially when there are large datasets. As nurses and midwives document large volumes, it is unsurprising that AI has potential to positively impact them. Indeed, there is great hope for what AI can offer nurses and midwives.

The guidelines and consensus statements on AI in nursing offer examples of where nurses could benefit from AI. This includes the ability to support delivery of evidence-based person-centred care, building stronger knowledge base for nursing, and removing mundane tasks that may potentially release time to care (Ronquillo et al. 2021). However, the consensus statements also concluded that to maximise the use of AI, nurses need to engage more with AI-related discussions, bridge gaps in knowledge about the data collected and get involved in AI from development to implementation. It also called for more work to understand the opportunity AI could offer nursing (Ronquillo et al. 2021). This suggests that there are still many unknowns about how AI could impact nursing. This will change as digitisation of health services continues and digital maturity increases.

More recently, in a scoping literature review of the evidence of AI in nursing, von Gerick et al. (2022) discovered that contemporary research on use of AI in nursing covered the initial stages of technology development, rather than its implementation or impact on practice. The work determined that most of the published studies of AI were focused on predictive modelling. There was a range of nursing activities where AI was being used, including care planning, risk prediction and documentation. Areas of interest included pressure ulcers, wound management, falls, deterioration, pain and infection management. Many of these areas of focus are associated with nursing care and nurse sensitive outcomes. Although it is good to see this work developing, it also demonstrates that there is more to do to move the use of AI from development to mainstream application. Only when this happens is there likely to be a significant impact on nurses and midwives.

When discussing predictive analytics, machine learning and AI, it is essential to call out the need to be aware of potential risks to health equity. Nurses/midwives need to remain cognizant of this potential bias when algorithms are developed, tested, and implemented. Not defining the problem fully, using poor-quality data or only some of the data needed to address the problem are areas where issues commonly arise (Roberts 2019). Being aware that the quality of good data is key should help ensure that the data used is strong enough. There is also a need to clinically validate the algorithm, understand underlying assumptions used and continually monitor initial use. To be able to support this effectively, nurses and midwives need to be part of the development team. This requires equipping nurses and midwives with a basic understanding of AI and its application, and supporting them to get and stay involved. To many, this may sound complex and technical. However, Roberts (2019), in an article exploring how AI and robots are changing the nursing role, sets out the contribution of nurses in an AI team and the types of questions nurses might consider. This practical approach recognises the unique contribution of nurses and midwives to validate complex algorithms.

Voice Recognition

Studies suggest that speech recognition technology (voice to text) can speed up and enhance nursing documentation (Fratzke et al. 2014; Monica 2018). Medical professionals have used this technology for radiology reporting for many years, and there is much to be learnt from this. However, there are some limitations that may be more relevant to nursing and midwifery. For instance, it may be hard to use voice recognition effectively in a room with multiple patients all listening in and with background noise. By contrast, it may work well in clinics rooms and in single rooms which are quieter. The crucial element for anyone using this technology is to remember to read what is recorded on the computer screen, edit, spell check, and validate the entry for accuracy before finalising it as a permanent record.

Wearables and Ambient Monitoring

Wearables are becoming increasingly used in healthcare. In the UK, there is a high focus on wearables to provide monitoring of those who no longer need hospital care but still need monitoring as they recover at home in 'virtual' wards. The technology commonly used includes oxygen saturation and blood pressure monitoring. People with long-term conditions, such as diabetes, also use wearable devices to track blood sugar over time, showing a broader perspective than single ad hoc tests. From a nursing and midwifery perspective, being able to monitor key data brings new opportunities and challenges. Opportunities include being able to support data-driven triage more effectively and shape new models of care, such as virtual services. Challenges include individual ability to use the technology, accuracy, ownership, and use of the data, and responsibilities and accountability issues when longitudinal data is shared, especially if there are extended periods between healthcare appointments and data continues to be uploaded but is not reviewed. The question commonly asked is: What if the data shows something to be wrong but this was missed? Who is responsible? Currently, there is no definitive legal position on these issues in the UK.

Nurses and midwives have a role that includes educating and supporting patients to self-manage their health conditions. It would seem sensible to include the use of technology as part of this. In practical terms, it is important to record where the data came from and use professional judgement when using it.

In the future, technology will move beyond traditional voice recognition and wearables into ambient monitoring, an emerging technology that uses minimal or contactless sensors in a clinical space, that are sensitive to the person occupying that space, in combination with EHRs. The sensors could include camera, voice, movement, vital sign monitors, and/or thermal imaging. Haque et al. (2020) undertook a review to explore how ambient technology could shine light in hospital and daily living spaces. This work found that hospital case studies focused on mobilisation, infection control activities, surgical skills assessment, automated surgical count, and real-time documentation using voice to text whilst undertaking a patient assessment. In home living spaces, they identified research focused on functional needs assessment of a person and falls. There was also work in mental health, exploring symptom screening. Much of this work saw the move away from traditional ways of collecting data, such as patient self-reporting or clinician-led assessment, to using technology to collect objective data. Haque et al. (2020) concluded that ambient intelligence could offer a new way of healthcare delivery. However, Haque et al. (2020) also called out the need for further exploration of the social, legal and ethical issues associated with ambient monitoring, including privacy, fairness and transparency, alongside the regulatory and research ethics for this type of research.

For nurses/midwives, ambient monitoring could provide rich data about a person and their behaviours or physical condition, without the need to enter the room. This may be useful if the person is at risk of self-harm, risk of falls or risk of deterioration, to name but a few. The potential volume of data generated without the need for direct face-to-face contact is vast, and more than a human could generate in a traditional assessment. As such, ambient monitoring has the potential to give a richer perspective and reduce documentation burden, allowing nurses and midwives to spend more time using data for decision making and actions. It is also clear from the work of Haque et al. (2020) that there is a need for more research to be able to assess effectiveness and the impact of ambient technologies. This could mean it is some time before such technologies are mainstreamed. However, nurses and midwives are in a prime position to be able to undertake and support further research on this.

Patient-Entered Data

Increasingly, people are being encouraged to contribute to their health records. This may be through a patient portal, where they can update items such as medication, allergies or contact details, through a link sent seeking information as part of pre-visit assessment, or by digitally transferring data from a devise they have at home.

The person is, in most cases, the most under-utilised member of the multi-disciplinary team, so this is a big step forward to making sure their voice is heard. It can also help address issues such as data accuracy, as there is a personal stake to make sure that what is written is accurate. However, for many professionals, this can be a different way of working and requires support to change working practices and use the information provided by patients (Balsdon 2021). The support needed can range from encouragement to re-designing clinical pathways to optimise the use of person entered data.

Nurses and midwives are well placed to support and guide people and patients to contribute to, make sense of, and use the information in their healthcare records to self-manage. However, there is a need for nurses and midwives to change the ways they work so that they use and respond to the information provided. It requires having an open attitude to change as access to portals and adoption rates increase. However, it should also be remembered that a portal can only do so much, and good verbal communication skills will still be required.

MANAGING LARGE DATA SETS

These developments contribute to significant growth in the volume of data accessible to nurses and midwives. However, it adds complexity and specialist skills are required to utilise big datasets effectively. This is where data science and data scientists come in!

Data science seeks to extract knowledge and insights from data using scientific methods, data mining, machine learning and AI on big datasets. This aims to provide practice insights and support effective decision making (Subrahmanya et al. 2022). Data scientists are the experts that undertake this.

To harness this opportunity, nurses and midwives need to build great relationships with data scientists. This might seem simplistic, but this relationship will be crucial if the professions are to harness the opportunities and benefits that technology can offer in the long term. However, this is not a one-way relationship. As much as nurses/midwives need the scientists, data scientists also need access to the clinical workforce to help identify where they can have most impact for the long-term sustainability of healthcare.

CASE STUDY

Cambridge University Hospitals: Making the transition from nurse collected data to digitally generated data for the ward to board assurance framework.

Cambridge University Hospitals implemented an enterprise-wide EHR in 2014, having previously been paper based.

Following this, nurse leaders sought to make the transition from manual collection of nursing quality indicators to electronically generated indicators to inform near real-time clinical dashboards.

Nursing quality indicators were the way in which quality of care was assessed and monitored across the organisation, from ward to hospital board. The ambition was to release nurses from data collection whilst still generating meaningful information to enable and motivate nurses to change their practice toward using data for improvement.

CASE STUDY—cont'd

The manual collection involved a senior nurse from each inpatient ward reviewing five sets of case notes each week. This information was then sent to the audit department to complete data entry and then the business intelligence team to collate and upload so that the information was available for review each month. This process took an average of 5 weeks.

The new process did not require nurses to do anything other than document accurately in structured fields within the EHR. The business intelligence team automated the data flow from the EHR into clinical dashboards, enabling the data to be viewed at patient, ward, department, and organisation-wide levels. The data set reflected 100% of the patients admitted to the hospital.

Moving from paper to electronic nursing metrics was a momentous change that enabled the organisation to focus on measuring what was important to make meaningful improvements to care. Inefficiencies associated with paper-based data collection were reduced and nursing time on administrative work was released to care.

The outcomes seen as results of the change included:
- Changed attitudes and behaviours towards data. Nurses and midwives spent less time challenging the data and more time focusing on responding to the data. Consequently, safety and compliance improved.
- Streamlined data collection of objective data and improved data quality by reducing risk of auditor error and subjectivity of the assessor.
- Released 56 hours a week of nursing time from administrative work to care.

Conclusion

Nurses and midwives generate a large volume of data when they document the care they give. Technology enables them to move away from traditional data entry and collection to using data to drive improvement.

In this chapter, we explored how nursing and midwifery leaders use data, the types of data required for improvement projects, how data is evolving and the implications for practice. It also described data quality and qualities. For nurses and midwives to be able to harness digital technology and use this to drive improvement, they must have the knowledge and skills to practice and lead in a digitally enabled environment. This may require changes to the way in which they practice, document, and use data. The changes include using more structured data, validating digitally generated data, increasing knowledge and skills to analyse and interpret data and managing data securely.

LEARNING EXERCISES

- Describe the data culture in your organisation.
- How can you ensure that you and your team generate quality data?
- Make a list of the data you need to inform an improvement project you are leading and consider how you will obtain this.
- Describe your organisation's current state to incorporate digital data into practice and what actions you can take to optimise this.
- Find what data science and/or data experts you have in your organisation. Talk to them about the services they offer and the work you are undertaking to understand how they can help you!

Key Points

1. Data used should be of a high quality and this starts at the point of recording care. Good data in an EHR will mean that the quality of extracted data is equally good.
2. The data used for improvement should fit the purpose. It can be tempting to use existing data or data that can be extracted from digital systems; however, this may not be what is needed to understand the improvement (Just because you can collect it does not mean you should!).
3. All data should be kept secure, in and out of the EHR.
4. Subject matter help should be sought from, for example, data scientists, to support good analysis and interpretation of data and to use the data to drive improvement.
5. Professional judgement should be used, as the computer is not always right!

References

Balsdon, H., 2021. Introducing a digital portal that enables patients to access their health records. Nurs. Manag. 28 (6), 36–42. https://doi.org/10.7748/nm.2021.1994.

Collins, S., Couture, B., Kang, M.J., et al., 2018. Quantifying and visualizing nursing flow-sheet documentation burden in acute and critical care. AMIA Annu. Symp. Proc. 2018, 348–357.

Fratzke, J., Tucker, S., Shedenhelm, H., et al., 2014. Enhancing nursing practice by utilizing voice recognition for direct documentation. J. Nurs. Adm. 44 (2), 79–86. https://doi.org/10.1097/NNA.0000000000000030.

Government Data Hub, 2021. What Is Data Quality? Available at: https://www.gov.uk/government/news/what-is-data-quality.

Haque, A., Milstein, A., Fei-Fei, L., 2020. Illuminating the dark spaces of healthcare with ambient intelligence. Nature. 585, 193–202. https://doi.org/10.1038/s41586-020-2669-y.

Langley, G.J., Moen, R.D., Nolan, K.M., et al., 2009. The Improvement Guide. A Practical Approach to Enhancing Organizational Performance, second ed. Jossey-Bass, San Francisco.

McCarthy, J., 1956. What Is Artificial Intelligence? Stanford University. Available at: http://jmc.stanford.edu/artificial-intelligence/what-is-ai/index.html.

Monica, K., 2018. Using EHR Voice Recognition to Improve Clinical Documentation, Useability. Xtelligent Healthcare Media. Available at: https://ehrintelligence.com/news/using-ehr-voice-recognition-to-improve-clinical-documentation-usability.

NHS Digital, 2022. Information Standards. Available at: https://digital.nhs.uk/data-and-information/information-standards.

NHS England, 2015. Interoperability Handbook. Available at: https://www.england.nhs.uk/publication/interoperabilty-handbk/.

Roberts, N., 2019. How artificial intelligence is changing nursing. Nurs. Manag. 50 (9), 30–39. https://doi.org/10.1097/01.NUMA.0000578988.56622.21.

Ronquillo, C.E., Peltonen, L., Pruinelli, L., et al., 2021. Artificial intelligence in nursing: priorities and opportunities for a n international invitational think tanks of the nursing and artificial leadership collaborative. J. Adv. Nurs. 77 (9), 3707–3717. https://doi.org/10.1111/jan.14855.

Shah, A., 2019. Using data for improvement. Br. Med. J. 364, I189. https://doi.org/10.1136/bmj.l189.

Stacey, G., Westwood, G., 2022. Leadership Development for Nurses and Midwives. Elsevier, India.

Subrahmanya, S.V., Shetty, D.K., Patil, V., et al., 2022. The role of data science in healthcare advancements: applications, benefits and future prospects. Inter. J. Med. Sci. 191, 1473–1483. https://doi.org/10.1007/s11845-021-02730-z.

The King's Fund, 2022. Interoperability Is More than Technology. Available at: https://www.kingsfund.org.uk/publications/digital-interoperability-technology.

von Gerick, H., Moen, H., Block, L.J., et al., 2022. Artificial Intelligence -based technologies in nursing: a scoping literature review of the evidence. Int. J. Nurs. Stud. 127, 104153. https://doi.org/10.1016/j.ijnurstu.2021.104153.

CHAPTER 14

Harnessing Digital Technology to Provide Research Evidence for Nursing and Midwifery Practice

Laura-Maria Peltonen ■ Siobhan O'Connor ■ Aaron Conway ■ Nicholas R. Hardiker ■ Betina Ross S. Idnay ■ Charlene Ronquillo

LEARNING OUTCOMES

At the end of this chapter, the nurses will be able to:

- Recognise how data derived from digital tools can enhance the scientific evidence base for healthcare.
- Identify how digital tools and techniques can support nursing research.
- Understand the role of nurses in enabling research through digital practice.

Introduction

Scientific research can bring new knowledge to support clinical and managerial decision making in healthcare. This involves collecting, storing, processing and analysing health data from one or more sources, such as unwell individuals, their families, health and care professionals and people working in management or government. The move from paper-based patient and administrative records to digital health datasets, along with the provision of more digital health services, is creating new datasets that can be used for research. This change in the way data is utilised presents new research opportunities for nurses to help understand how patient care and health service delivery can be improved.

Furthermore, nurses are starting to use more technologies in their daily practice, such as electronic health records (EHRs) and clinical decision support systems (CDSS) (Booth et al. 2021). Patients and their families can also employ a range of technologies to support self-management at home, such as mobile applications (apps), telehealth and telecare, and online health services. Research can also be used to evaluate digitally enabled nursing and midwifery practice and digital forms of self-care.

This chapter considers the importance of health data generated through a range of digital technologies and examines how this can be used in nursing research. It discusses the tools and techniques for collecting and analysing digital data for health research, and how nurses in their everyday practice can apply the knowledge this generates. Finally, it discusses the role of nurses in using research to evaluate digitally enabled practice.

GENERATING HEALTH DATA VIA DIGITAL TECHNOLOGIES

Many technologies that nurses interact with, from EHRs to the medical devices that measure a person's physiological status, create a wealth of data about frontline care delivery. In addition, nurse managers can use digital tools and computerised systems to monitor and report issues, from patient safety to quality of care and staffing levels, generating more data on health service delivery. Patients can use technologies, such as mobile health applications and wearable devices, to self-manage illnesses at home or in care homes or to maintain their physical and mental health. Data from these digital technologies can be collected and stored in two main ways to enable future research.

First, it can be captured and stored as structured data, categorised in a particular standardised format that can be relatively fast and simple to understand. For example, a blood pressure reading will have specific measures (i.e. diastolic and systolic readings captured numerically) or a pain scale where a person's level of pain is documented from zero to ten. Checkboxes on an assessment form, along with diagnostic procedures and treatments, can be captured as structured data, as they have a specific value or meaning that are clear and easy to recognise. An instance of patient-generated structured data would be heart rate and step count collected via a fitness tracker.

Structured data that come in standardised formats can be gathered and analysed more easily by different digital tools and integrated with datasets in existing computer systems, making it more accessible for future research use. Persell et al. (2018) tested a medication management tool delivered through an EHR to see if it could help people with hypertension who visited community health centres. Their study found that the EHR tool improved medication reconciliation and, when combined with nurse-led support, it enhanced participants' understanding of medication instructions and dosing.

Second, it can be captured and stored as unstructured data, that is, free-text and descriptive notes that nurses may record about the people in their care, which can be more complicated and take more time to understand. For example, a description of a wound, such as a pressure ulcer or a care plan explaining the types of care delivered to an individual each day. An instance of patient-generated unstructured data could be health-related content (e.g. written text, images, audio or video) added by the patient into the EHR or posted on social media platforms, such as Facebook, Twitter, Instagram, or YouTube.

Unstructured data consisting of rich narratives that detail the complexity of a person's health and care can be more challenging to collect and analyse via digital technologies, making it less accessible for research use. However, newer analytical techniques that involve labelling unstructured datasets and employing computational linguistics are being developed to help with this. Nakatani et al. (2020)

used artificial intelligence (AI) techniques, such as machine learning and Natural Language Processing (NLP), to identify risk factors and create a predictive model on the likelihood of hospital falls based on nursing records extracted from an EHR. From this study, a falls risk monitoring system could be developed to support nurses to identify people at risk of falling and put strategies in place to prevent this. Despite the different types and formats of health data that can be collected via technology, the availability of vast amounts of digital data is enabling nurses to undertake health research that could improve care.

THE QUALITY OF HEALTH DATA

Health data gathered in both paper and digital forms can vary in quality. There are several characteristics of data quality (DQ) that are important to consider, as they can affect frontline care as well as the conduct and reporting of health research. Fadahunsi et al. (2021) identified three dimensions and 13 measures of data quality in relation to digital health technologies, many of which are applicable to nursing research and practice (Table 14.1). For example, accuracy may be compromised if a person's full blood count (FBC) data is recorded in the wrong record or entered in the correct record but with the wrong date. Data security may be affected if digital tools do not have robust forms of authentication and authorisation. Hence,

TABLE 14.1 ■ **Characteristics of Data Quality in Healthcare**

DQ Dimension	DQ Measure	Description
Informativeness	Accuracy	How much the information is correct
	Completeness	How much the information is complete/missing
	Interpretability	How much the information can be understood
	Plausibility	How much the information makes sense based on common knowledge
	Provenance	How much the information source is trustworthy
	Relevance	How much the information is useful for a set task
Availability	Accessibility	How much the information is easy to obtain
	Portability	How much the information is accessible in different systems
	Security	How much the information is protected from unauthorised access or exploitation
	Timeliness	How much current information is available on time
Usability	Conformance	How much information is in a desired format
	Consistency	How much information is in the same format
	Maintainability	How much information can be maintained

Adapted from Fadahunsi et al. (2021).

developing and implementing data management plans to ensure the privacy, security, and confidentiality of health data is paramount in nursing research, so that all relevant data protection policies and legislation are adhered to.

When data is collected retrospectively from historical health records, which is the most common approach when undertaking research, the quality of the digital dataset must be taken into consideration, as errors or omissions can affect the analysis and findings of research. For example, nurses typically document only 'clinically relevant' data, while other data (e.g. socio-economic, cultural and political) are not typically found in EHRs. Furthermore, a review of a national hospital registry containing longitudinal data on over seven million patients found that different coding and classification systems for diagnostics and treatments changed over several years, leaving some records incomplete or inconsistent (Schmidt et al. 2015). When data collection is planned in advance and the data gathered in real-time, the quality can be affected by the time, research expertise, funding and other resources needed to collect, process or clean, store and analyse digital health data. Password-protected databases are often used to securely store digital health data.

As these types of electronic datasets are used extensively for health research, a number of validation techniques should be used when processing digital health data to prevent age, gender, race or other biases that could lead to flawed research results. Feder (2018) outlined a range of statistical methods that can account for aspects of poor data quality in EHRs. Moreover, a thorough understanding of the context and format of digital data is also important, as it can affect the generation and use of scientific evidence. For instance, Rusanov et al. (2014) highlighted a potential bias towards those who are more unwell when choosing research participants from EHRs, as more laboratory and medication data is captured regarding these individuals, making them more likely to be included in research. Therefore, educating nurses about the importance of data quality in digital health technologies and providing organisational infrastructure and training on approaches to improve this, along with upskilling in database management techniques (e.g. structured query language [SQL] programming), could lead to more robust and accurate research that informs professional practice (Peltonen et al. 2019).

ANALYSING DIGITAL HEALTH DATA

A range of digital tools support the analysis and understanding of digital health data used in nursing research. Common software packages include SPSS, which is used to analyse quantitative (including categorical) data gathered via surveys or questionnaires or extracted from EHRs. For example, different types of descriptive and inferential statistics can be run using SPSS to generate the mean, median, standard deviation, p-value, confidence interval, odds ratio, as well as other analyses. This can provide insights about the incidence or prevalence of conditions, or if a digital intervention, such as a mobile application has a positive, negative or neutral effect on a person's health. For example, Sittig et al. (2020) assessed if a mobile app could help people with diabetes change their behaviour. They analysed user metrics on the app to show that it improved self-efficacy and exercise and could improve health-related behaviours.

NVivo (https://lumivero.com/products/nvivo/) is a popular software package used to analyse qualitative data (written text or transcribed audio) that can be collected via interviews, focus groups or documentation (e.g. nursing or midwifery notes or care plans) extracted from EHRs and other hospital or primary care computer systems. NVivo supports nurse researchers in electronically coding and categorising the complexity of health data that is qualitative in nature, so general trends or themes in the digital dataset can be identified and subsequently, inform practice. For instance, O'Connor et al. (2018) used Microsoft Excel and NVivo to analyse the content of tweets from a Twitter chat on multi-morbidity led by a group of senior clinical nurses. They reported a number of key challenges, including supporting people to cope with treatment burden, delivering holistic care, re-designing health services and developing a stronger evidence base on those with multiple long-term conditions.

More advanced forms of analysis can be conducted on qualitative data using machine learning and NLP, two domains within AI. However, this requires specialised programming expertise in languages such as Python and R. Therefore, nurses may benefit from collaborating with colleagues in the computer science and data science departments if more complex analysis, predictive modelling and data visualisations are required, particularly if the final research output is likely to be integrated into clinical IT systems in the future to improve the quality of care and patient outcomes.

EVALUATING DIGITALLY ENABLED PRACTICE VIA RESEARCH

Digital technologies provide new opportunities to optimise clinical workflows and improve care. However, using technology involves numerous interactions between different health professionals, health service managers, administrators and others who use digital tools, such as CDSSs and EHRs within complex working environments. Sometimes, barriers can exist to introducing new technologies in clinical practice or they can have unintended consequences (e.g. professional burnout or impaired decision making) if the hardware or software is not designed to fit the way nurses work. Therefore, it is important to design digital tools robustly and with the involvement of nurses, and to evaluate their impact via scientific research to assess if they have a positive effect on nursing practice (Booth et al. 2021).

For example, research studies have conducted usability evaluations of digital tools like EHRs and mobile apps to understand how they affect the performance of physicians, nurses, midwives and other healthcare professionals, patient outcomes, and why they choose to adopt or abandon them (Persell et al. 2018). Research has also explored organisational level issues when introducing new technologies, such as electronic prescribing systems, to understand the factors that lead to the success or failure of this type of change. Hence, research on all aspects of digitally enabled nursing practice is critical to evaluate whether digital technologies are worth investing in and to understand how they should be designed and deployed within an organisational setting to bring about positive change in clinical practice.

LEARNING EXERCISE

Read the following example of how data is collected and used in Finland and answer the questions below:

In Finland hospitals, nurses' documentation of care is done based on the nursing process into EHRs. The documentation is based on standardised terminologies and has structured formats as well as unstructured nursing narratives. This collection of data enables nursing leadership to monitor delivered services. Examples include nursing sensitive outcomes such as pressure ulcers, pain care, patient falls, and nosocomial infections.

The Finnish 'National Peer Development in Nursing' project is one example, where a system has been created for measuring, producing, evaluating and developing the quality of nursing. A national consortium of experts from the field has identified key indicators and built a system, which is embedded into the quality monitoring work of social and healthcare organisations. The information collected supports the allocation of operational resources on organisational levels to improve service delivery, patient safety and operational effectiveness. Additionally, the systematic monitoring of information regarding the quality on nursing work can be presented to service users, researchers and policy makers.

1. What do you think the benefits are to nursing practice and research of having structured data about nursing assessments, interventions and outcomes?
2. What types of questions could be addressed using a country-wide EHR system that has nursing data?

CASE STUDY

Early detection of patients' risk for deterioration is crucial to provide relevant interventions that could help prevent inpatient deaths caused by cardiac arrest and sepsis. Despite clinicians' best efforts to deliver the highest quality of care, the challenges in timely inter-professional communication between nurses and doctors can cause delays in patient treatment. When nurses notice subtle yet concerning changes in a patient's physiological condition, they frequently boost patient surveillance and EHR documentation for those patients. By incorporating an early warning system into EHRs, hospitals would have a means of alerting the inter professional team to any growing nursing concerns about alterations in patient states. The COmmunicating Narrative Concerns Entered by RNs (CONCERN) clinical decision support system (CDSS) was developed by nursing researchers in the United States to predict and provide clinical decision support when patients are at an increased risk of deterioration. The CONCERN CDDS analyses the trends in nursing documentation that represent nursing surveillance and suggest nurses' shifting levels of concern. A preliminary study indicated that the system was able to detect patient deterioration 42 hours earlier than existing deterioration scoring methods. The CONCERN CDDS is currently being evaluated in a large research study to test for effectiveness and usability (Rossetti et al. 2021). It is a good example of how nurses can develop digital interventions to improve care using data from an EHR, and how these are then evaluated in a research study.

https://www.nursingworld.org/foundation/rninitiative/technology-enabled-nursing-practice/concern-implementation-toolkit/

Conclusion

This chapter discusses how digital technologies and the data they generate can be used to support research into nursing practice. It provides an overview of the advantages and disadvantages of structured and unstructured health datasets and outlines the key aspects of data quality that are important to capture in digital systems, as this can influence the findings and applicability of research evidence. The complexities of capturing health data retrospectively or prospectively are also considered along with these types of digital data that can impact the generation and reporting of nursing research.

Importantly, the approaches used for analysing a range of digital data are discussed so that nurses can develop their expertise in statistical and other analytical methods to generate high-quality health research. Finally, the value of evaluating digitally enabled nursing practice through robust scientific research is highlighted, as digital tools are multi-faceted interventions rolled out within complex organisations involving numerous stakeholders which can bring benefits, risks, and limitations. Hence, more research into how to design and implement digital tools with nurses in hospital and community settings would enable the collection of better-quality digital datasets, which could be utilised to improve care.

Key Points

1. Nurses generate valuable health data that should be digitised so that it can be used more easily to conduct research and support professional practice and patient care.
2. Systematic methods when collecting and analysing digital health data should be developed to enhance data quality, facilitating accurate interpretation that benefits care.
3. Training should be provided to nurses to upskill them in using a range of technologies and the digital health datasets they generate.
4. Robust research into designing and deploying technologies in healthcare is needed to ensure that the digitally enabled practice of nurses actually improves care.
5. Further education that supports nurses to conduct digital health research should be delivered to drive innovation and lead to the creation, introduction, and evaluation of new technologies that could benefit frontline care and the delivery of health services.

References

Booth, R.G., Strudwick, G., McBride, S., et al., 2021. How the nursing profession should adapt for a digital future. BMJ. 373. https://doi.org/10.1136/bmj.n1190.

Fadahunsi, K.P., O'Connor, S., Akinlua, J.T., et al., 2021. Information quality frameworks for digital health technologies: systematic review. J. Med. Internet Res. 23 (5), e23479. https://doi.org/10.2196/23479.

Feder, S.L., 2018. Data quality in electronic health records research: quality domains and assessment methods. West. J. Nurs. Res. 40 (5), 753–766. https://doi.org/10.1177/0193945916689084.

Nakatani, H., Nakao, M., Uchiyama, H., et al., 2020. Predicting inpatient falls using natural language processing of nursing records obtained from Japanese electronic medical records: case-control study. JMIR Med. Inf. 8 (4), e16970. https://doi.org/10.2196/16970.

O'Connor, S., Deaton, C., Nolan, F., et al., 2018. Nursing in an age of multimorbidity. BMC Nurs. 17 (1). https://doi.org/10.1186/s12912-018-0321-z.

Peltonen, L.M., Nibber, R., Lewis, A., et al., 2019. Emerging professionals' observations of opportunities and challenges in nursing informatics. Nurs. Leader. 32 (2), 8–18. https://doi.org/10.12927/cjnl.2019.25965.

Persell, S.D., Karmali, K.N., Lazar, D., et al., 2018. Effect of electronic health record–based medication support and nurse-led medication therapy management on hypertension and medication self-management: a randomized clinical trial. JAMA Intern. Med. 178 (8), 1069–1077. https://doi.org/10.1001/jamainternmed.2018.2372.

Rossetti, S.C., Dykes, P.C., Knaplund, C., et al., 2021. The communicating narrative concerns entered by registered nurses (CONCERN) clinical decision support early warning system: protocol for a cluster randomized pragmatic clinical trial. JMIR Res. Protoc. 10 (12), e30238. https://doi.org/10.2196/30238.

Rusanov, A., Weiskopf, N.G., Wang, S., et al., 2014. Hidden in plain sight: bias towards sick patients when sampling patients with sufficient electronic health record data for research. BMC Med. Inf. Decis. Making. 14 (51). https://doi.org/10.1186/1472-6947-14-51.

Schmidt, M., Schmidt, S.A.J., Sandegaard, J.L., et al., 2015. The Danish national patient registry: a review of content, data quality, and research potential. Clin. Epidemiol. 7, 449–490.

Sittig, S., Wang, J., Iyengar, S., et al., 2020. Incorporating behavioral trigger messages into a mobile health app for chronic disease management: randomized clinical feasibility trial in diabetes. JMIR MHealth UHealth. 8 (3), e15927. https://doi.org/10.2196/15927.

The Future Potential for Digitally Enabled Person-Centred Practice

SECTION OUTLINE

CHAPTER 15

Artificial Intelligence in Nursing

Siobhan O'Connor

Introduction

Artificial intelligence (AI) is a term used to describe a range of advanced computational techniques developed and applied to digital datasets in an attempt to mimic aspects of human intelligence. This can include elements such as abstract reasoning, learning, decision-making, and communicating or interacting with a physical or virtual world. Samoili et al. (2020: 4) define AI as:

> software (and possibly also hardware) systems designed by humans that, given a complex goal, act in the physical or digital dimension by perceiving their environment through data acquisition, interpreting the collected structured or unstructured data, reasoning on the knowledge, or processing the information, derived from this data and deciding the best action(s) to take to achieve the given goal. AI systems can either use symbolic rules or learn a numeric model, and they can also adapt their behaviour by analysing how the environment is affected by their previous actions.

AI can analyse any type of data, including written text, audio (voice) data, as well as visual data from images and videos or a combination of these data. The most common set of AI approaches is called machine learning techniques that are used to predict events and help with diagnosis, for example. Machine learning is made up of many different types of algorithms that build mathematical models based on data to make predictions or decisions. An early example of this in nursing can be seen in a study by Harvey (1993), who used a neural network to support the nursing diagnostic process. Another popular AI approach is called natural language processing

(NLP), which uses a range of computation techniques to break down words and phrases in sentences and paragraphs to understand what they mean. However, it is important to know there are other computational approaches in the AI field and people continue to research and develop new techniques and apply them in different ways.

Algorithms, which are a set of software instructions used to process data and perform calculations, are used in machine learning, NLP, and other areas in AI. Some of these algorithms are also used in neighbouring fields, such as data science, text mining and traditional statistics (Russell et al. 2022). Hence, there is some overlap between the four domains of AI, data science, text mining and statistics as they share some techniques (Figure 15.1). This chapter considers the importance of algorithms in analysing and understanding digital health data and AI-based tools that can be used in nursing practice. It discusses the computational techniques that can be used for analysing digital data in nursing research, and how nurses in their everyday practice can adopt and use AI-based technologies in professional practice. Finally, it discusses the limitations and risks of AI in healthcare and the role of nurses in utilising AI to support digitally enabled practice.

Analysing Digital Health Data Via AI Techniques

The main set of AI techniques is called machine learning. These algorithms are categorised in three ways:

(1) supervised learning
(2) unsupervised learning
(3) reinforcement learning

First, in supervised machine learning, a subset of the digital dataset needs to be annotated or labelled by a human expert. This is called the training dataset and the labels are associated with specific data variables (features). For example, if you

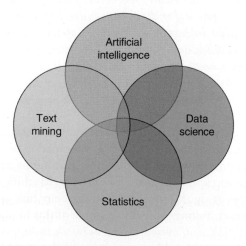

Fig. 15.1 Domains that share some computational techniques with AI.

have a wound care dataset and you wish to understand which wounds are at risk of infection, you might label certain words or phrases such as 'slough' and 'exudate' as being related to infection. Then, you may utilise one or more algorithms to help build a mathematical model based on the labelled or 'training' dataset, which is usually 20%–30% of the overall dataset (Russell et al. 2022). The algorithm learns rules or trends in the training dataset based on the labelled data and then applies these to the larger test dataset, which generates the final predictive output or model. Some common supervised machine learning algorithms include decision tree and random forest, each of which is designed to analyse data in a specific way (Table 15.1). An example of these types of AI algorithms is observed in a study by Hirdes et al. (2008), who developed and applied a decision tree algorithm to help prioritise access to care home services for older adults. They used a dataset of over 4000 older adults to identify factors that predict nursing home placement. Then, they created a computerised decision support tool based on the algorithm to help case managers identify people at risk or at high need of care homes services.

One of the most popular supervised machine learning techniques is called artificial neural network (ANN), where data is processed through layers. This algorithm comprises layers of nodes, containing an input layer, one or more hidden layers in the middle, and an output layer at the end; this is why it is often referred to as 'deep learning' (Figure 15.2). Each node is made up of inputs, weights, a threshold, and an output. If an output value exceeds the threshold, the node is activated and data is passed to the next layer in the network (Gupta et al. 2021). As there can be many layers in a neural network, it is not possible to identify which variables in the dataset were used by the algorithm to arrive at the predicted outcome or model. Hence, they are often referred to as a 'black box'. As with all supervised learning techniques, this algorithm relies on training data to learn and improve its accuracy over time, which can help it classify and cluster large volumes of data at high speed. There are many different types of neural networks (e.g. perceptrons, convolutional and recurrent) as they can be set up or configured in different ways for different purposes. ANNs are used frequently in healthcare to analyse medical images. For instance, Jain et al. (2021) developed a web-based tool and used photographs of skin conditions and patients' medical history to build a predictive model based on an ANN to improve the identification of skin conditions in primary care where dermatological expertise can be limited.

The second category of machine learning is called unsupervised learning. These algorithms work differently as they are used to analyse and cluster unlabelled datasets to discover patterns or data groupings without the need for human intervention. These types of algorithms are used for different tasks, such as clustering, association rules, and dimensionality reduction (to reduce noise or variance in a dataset if it is too big without losing data integrity). There are numerous different algorithms in this category, such as K-means clustering and Principal Component Analysis (PCA) (Table 15.1) (Celebi and Aydin 2016). An example of this in nursing can be seen in a study by An et al. (2021), who extracted data on 300 critical care patients from a hospital's electronic medical record system. They used a number of AI algorithms,

TABLE 15.1 ■ **Descriptions of Key AI Terms**

AI Term	Description
Algorithm	A set of software instructions that help solve a problem or perform a computation.
Artificial intelligence	Advanced computational techniques developed and applied to digital data to try to imitate aspects of human intelligence.
Artificial neural network	A type of machine learning algorithm where data are processed through layers (input layer, one or more hidden layers and an output layer).
Computer vision	A domain within artificial intelligence that uses machine learning algorithms to analyse digital visual data, such as photographs and videos.
Decision tree	A type of machine learning algorithm that breaks down a dataset into smaller subsets based on certain variables (features) in the dataset until a decision (prediction) is made.
K-means clustering	A type of machine learning algorithm used to cluster or group similar data together, as it partitions a dataset into a certain number of clusters.
Machine learning	A set of algorithms that build mathematical models based on data to make predictions or decisions.
Natural language processing	A range of computation techniques that break down words and phrases into sentences and paragraphs to understand what human language means.
Principal component analysis	A statistical technique used on a dataset with numerous variables (features) to reduce the number of features without affecting the quality of the dataset.
Random forest	A type of machine learning algorithm that combines multiple decision trees into a single model, where each tree is trained on a subset of a dataset and a subset of the variables (features); the algorithm combines the results of all the trees to make a prediction.

including K-means clustering, to assign patients into three sub-groups using 16 different characteristics: eight related to disease severity and eight to nursing workload. This approach could be used to help nurse managers identify similar patient groups who have specific care needs and then assign nursing staff according to their levels of clinical experience to improve the management of critically ill patients.

The third and last category of machine learning is called reinforcement learning. These algorithms work in a very different way, in that they optimise sequential decisions repeated over time in a dynamic system that operates under uncertainty; that

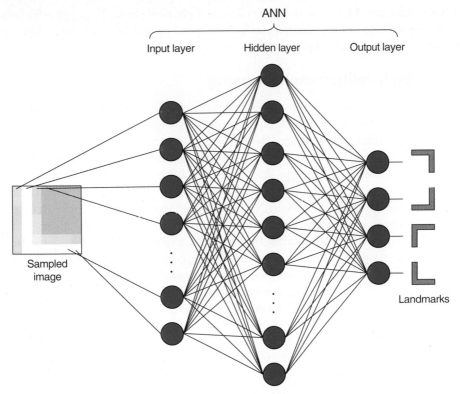

Fig. 15.2   A visualisation of an artificial neural network.

is, the real-world conditions. For instance, audio or text-based chatbots often use reinforcement learning techniques to learn how to respond to human users. These algorithms work within a mathematical framework that has three main elements: (1) a state space, which is the available information or problem features to work with; (2) an action space, which is the decisions algorithms can take at each state of the system; and (3) a reward signal, which is the feedback (positive or negative) algorithms receive on how it has performed. In healthcare, reinforcement learning algorithms have been used to customise email notifications sent to women using behavioural nudging techniques to encourage them to attend appointments for mammography screening (Bucher et al. 2022).

Lastly, NLP is another branch of AI that has its own set of computational linguistic techniques or symbolic rules to understand and respond to human language in text or voice form, particularly large unstructured datasets. NLP often combines traditional statistical techniques with machine learning algorithms and its own computational linguistic abilities (rule-based modelling of human language) to break down and understand text of voice data. It is being used in healthcare in many ways. For instance, Annapragada et al. (2021) employed several NLP techniques to analyse free-text notes about children's health from physicians, nurses, and social workers extracted from electronic medical records. This was used to train an

ANN to identify children at risk of or victims of physical abuse. This approach could be developed into a computerised platform to speed up and improve the accuracy of referring children to child protection services.

Artificial Intelligence in Nursing

A systematic review of AI in nursing identified 140 research studies that used machine learning and NLP techniques in various ways to analyse patient, administrative, and other health-related datasets (O'Connor et al. 2022). The most common clinical practice areas were critical care, wound care, falls, infection, and older adult care (Table 15.2). Various AI techniques have also been used in different areas of nursing administration and management to help predict nurse staffing in acute setting, levels of bullying, or burnout among nurses. Advanced computational techniques can also be applied to datasets in nursing education, as the review found a handful of studies that used AI to predict student dropout from undergraduate nursing programmes, and failure, completion and graduation rates. While many of the studies reported some potential benefits of using AI algorithms, most only developed and tested a number of algorithms on health datasets. They did not create any AI-based digital tool that could be used by nurses to support care or roll out an AI-based tool with practising nurses in a real-world health setting, such as a hospital. Therefore, how AI can affect the workflow and workload of nurses in different areas of professional practice remains unknown (O'Connor et al. 2022).

TABLE 15.2 ■ Areas of Nursing Where AI Techniques Have Been Employed

Area of Nursing	AI Techniques Applied
Critical care	Example: To investigate and compare physician and nursing notes, in the first 48 hours of admission, to predict ICU length of stay and mortality. Huang et al. 2021
Wound care	Example: To develop and assess the impact of a decision support intervention to predict hospital acquired pressure ulcers and on the user adoption rate and attitudes. Cho et al. 2013
Falls	Example: To develop fall risk prediction models using EMR data and to evaluate the predictive performance by comparing it to the Hendrich II Fall Risk Model Validation. Jung et al. 2020
Infection	Example: To discover knowledge about hospital-acquired catheter-associated urinary tract infections. Park et al. 2023
Older adult care	Example: To determine how well AI algorithms could accurately classify frailty against a calculated 36-item electronic frailty index. Ambagtsheer et al. 2020

PROBLEMS WITH ARTIFICIAL INTELLIGENCE

Although AI techniques can be useful to help understand complex data, there are several limitations and risks associated with algorithms. One of the biggest problems with AI at present is 'algorithmic bias', which can result from poor-quality datasets with missing information, as well as socio-demographic characteristics, such as age, gender and race, of certain groups of people. These missing data could introduce bias into predictive models, as it would result in AI techniques being trained on a dataset that does not fully represent the people of interest in a population, leading to widening health inequalities in some populations. Remember, AI is only as good as the dataset it is trained on. A landmark research in the United States identified racial bias in an algorithm used by a health insurance company to calculate who needed extra health-care, with black patients assigned the same level of risk as white patients, despite being more unwell (Obermeyer et al. 2019). Another concern with AI is that we do not fully understand how some of the algorithms work, such as knowing which variables (features) in the dataset are used to build a predictive model, often referred to as 'black box' AI. This lack of transparency can cause trust issues with AI-based tools, especially if how they work cannot be explained fully and they are being relied on to inform clinical and managerial decision-making. For example, an AI model that is designed to detect cancer, even if it is 99% accurate could still be life threatening for the 1% of cases that it potentially misses. Hence, clinical accountability and autonomy are important, and nurses and other professionals must interpret the results of a predictive model and combine it with clinical judgment and expertise to support decision-making and care delivery. Furthermore, calls for more transparency in how AI algorithms work may need to be balanced with security issues to prevent algorithms and the computer systems they are based on from being hacked by malicious actors. Therefore, the World Health Organization (2021) has outlined six principles to ensure AI is developed and applied appropriately to address some of its limitations and risks:

1) protecting human autonomy;
2) promoting human wellbeing and safety and the public interest;
3) ensuring transparency, explainability, and intelligibility;
4) fostering responsibility and accountability;
5) ensuring inclusiveness and equity and
6) promoting AI that is responsive and sustainable.

NURSES' ROLE IN ARTIFICIAL INTELLIGENCE

Nurses have an important role to play in the development, use, and evaluation of AI and AI-based technologies in healthcare to support digitally-enabled practice. To be able to do this, nurses need to be educated about this emerging area of informatics so they can engage with research and practice on AI-based digital tools (Booth et al. 2021; O'Connor et al. 2022). Some nurses may also benefit from specialist training to learn, in more depth, how machine learning and NLP work. Once nurses have some knowledge and skills in AI, they will be able to think of ways to utilise algorithms for nursing and other health datasets to help understand and solve some of the problems faced by the profession in acute hospital and community settings. Any ideas for AI-based digital tools could then be taken to internal colleagues working in information technology (IT) and data analytics or to external professionals working in computer science at a university or a commercial software company to turn an idea for an AI-based tool into reality. Another useful step would be for nurses to collaborate with clinical and managerial colleagues in the health service to develop an AI tool further, as the initiative will likely take a lot of time, money and multidisciplinary expertise to be successful. Finally, nurses should implement a new AI tool in a real-world environment and evaluate how well it works with nurses and patients. This would generate robust evidence on AI in nursing to support professional practice.

LEARNING EXERCISE

Read the following example of how data were collected and analysed using machine learning algorithms and answer the questions below:

In the United States, nurses use electronic health records (EHR) to document hospital-acquired pressure injuries that occur in critical care. The decision about which patient would benefit from a special pressure-relieving mattress can be difficult, as most critical care patients are at high risk. Machine learning techniques (e.g. random forest algorithm) could be used to develop a mathematical model that predicts the development of pressure ulcers using EHR data (e.g. age, vital signs, weight, mobility, skin condition and nutrition). If the model was relatively accurate and validated, it could be used to design a digital dashboard of metrics to inform nurses about people 'at risk' of developing a pressure ulcer while in hospital and who may be more suitable for speciality versus standard beds and mattresses. This could be utilised alongside or as an alternative to traditional assessment tools, such as the Braden Scale to prevent or reduce the occurrence of pressure injuries.
1. What do you think are the benefits to nurses when they have a more sophisticated way to identify patients at risk of pressure ulcers?
2. What might be a limitation or risk of using algorithms and AI tools to predict pressure injuries among people in hospital?

CASE STUDY

A new AI-based assessment tool called Mia™ is being developed by a UK company to analyse mammograms from screening programmes to improve the prediction of breast cancer. The tool uses a specific type of artificial neural network (deep learning) called a convoluted neural network to analyse a large dataset of over 3 million medical images from multiple hospitals. The plan is to use this new AI tool to speed up the screening and diagnosis process for women, so that radiologists do not have to double-check each individual mammogram but can use Mia™ instead as an automated assessment tool to support their initial clinical decision. Importantly, if the radiologist and the AI tool do not agree on the same diagnosis, then a second radiologist can be consulted for additional expertise.

https://transform.england.nhs.uk/ai-lab/explore-all-resources/understand-ai/mia-mammography-intelligent-assessment/.

Conclusion

This chapter discusses the main advanced computational techniques that comprise AI and the principles by which machine learning and NLP work. It provides an overview of how AI is being applied in nursing research and practice and outlines its benefits, limitations and risks. It also highlights some of the complexities of AI for the nursing profession, along with the impact algorithms and predictive modelling can have on frontline care and management of health services. Finally, nurses' role in AI in healthcare is emphasised in relation to education, innovation, collaboration and implementation to ensure the profession can capitalise on these new computational techniques and utilise them to understand health datasets and solve problems that nurses come across in their day-to-day practice.

Key Points

1. High quality nursing datasets should be collected via electronic means, and digital infrastructure, such as electronic health records and mobile devices, should be put in place to support this, which would enable more AI research and practice.
2. Nurses need education and training on predictive algorithms and other computational techniques in the AI field, so they can participate in and lead AI initiatives in healthcare.
3. Nurses should be more involved in applying AI algorithms to health datasets and in evaluating AI-based digital tools using rigorous scientific methods to ensure they are safe and improve care.
4. The ethical, social and legal implications of AI in nursing need more research so that robust AI-based digital tools that support professional practice and frontline care can be created.

References

Ambagtsheer, R.C., Shafiabady, N., Dent, E., et al., 2020. The application of artificial intelligence (AI) techniques to identify frailty within a residential aged care administrative data set. Int. J. Med. Inf. 136, 104094. https://doi.org/10.1016/j.ijmedinf.2020.104094.

An, R., Chang, G.M., Fan, Y.Y., et al., 2021. Machine learning–based patient classification system for adult patients in intensive care units: a cross–sectional study. J. Nurs. Manag. 29 (6), 1752–1762. https://doi.org/10.1111/jonm.13284.

Annapragada, A.V., Donaruma-Kwoh, M.M., Annapragada, A.V., et al., 2021. A natural language processing and deep learning approach to identify child abuse from pediatric electronic medical records. PLoS One. 16 (2), e0247404. https://doi.org/10.1371/journal.pone.0247404.

Booth R G, Strudwick G, McBride S, O'Connor S, Solano Lopez A L, 2021. How the nursing profession should adapt for a digital future. BMJ ; 373 :n1190 doi:10.1136/bmj.n1190

Bucher, A., Blazek, E.S., West, A.B., 2022. Feasibility of a reinforcement learning–enabled digital health intervention to promote mammograms: retrospective, single-arm, observational study. JMIR. Form. Res. 6 (11), e42343. https://doi.org/10.2196/42343.

Celebi, M.E., Aydin, K. (Eds.), 2016. Unsupervised Learning Algorithms. Springer, Cham. https://doi.org/10.1007/978-3-319-24211-8.

Cho, I., Park, I., Kim, E., et al., 2013. Using EHR data to predict hospital-acquired pressure ulcers: a prospective study of a Bayesian Network model. Int. J. Med. Inf. 82 (11), 1059–1067. https://doi.org/10.1016/j.ijmedinf.2013.06.012.

Gupta, D., Kose, U., Le Nguyen, B., et al. (Eds.), 2021. Artificial Intelligence for Data-Driven Medical Diagnosis. Walter de Gruyter GmbH, Berlin.

Harvey, R.M., 1993. Nursing diagnosis by computers: an application of neural networks. Int. J. Nurs. Terminol. Classif. 4 (1), 26–34. https://doi.org/10.1111/j.1744-618X.1993.tb000 80.x.

Hirdes, J.P., Poss, J.W., Curtin-Telegdi, N., 2008. The Method for Assigning Priority Levels (MAPLe): a new decision-support system for allocating home care resources. BMC Med. 6 (1), 1–11. https://doi.org/10.1186/1741-7015-6-9.

Huang, K., Gray, T.F., Romero-Brufau, S., et al., 2021. Using nursing notes to improve clinical outcome prediction in intensive care patients: a retrospective cohort study. J. Am. Med. Inf. Assoc. 28 (8), 1660–1666. https://doi.org/10.1093/jamia/ocab051.

Jain, A., Way, D., Gupta, V., et al., 2021. Development and assessment of an artificial intelligence–based tool for skin condition diagnosis by primary care physicians and nurse practitioners in teledermatology practices. JAMA Netw. Open 4 (4), e217249. https://doi.org/10.1001/jamanetworkopen.2021.7249.

Jung, H., Park, H.-A., Hwang, H., 2020. Improving prediction of fall risk using electronic health record data with various types and sources at multiple times. Comput. Inform. Nurs. 38 (3), 157–164. https://doi.org/10.1097/CIN.0000000000000561.

Obermeyer, Z., Powers, B., Vogeli, C., et al., 2019. Dissecting racial bias in an algorithm used to manage the health of populations. Science 366 (6464), 447–453. https://doi.org/10.11 26/science.aax2342.

O'Connor, S., Yan, Y., Thilo, F., et al., 2022. Artificial intelligence in nursing and midwifery: a systematic review. J. Clin. Nurs. Available at: https://doi.org/10.1111/jocn.16478.

Park, J.I., Bliss, D.Z., Chi, C.-L., et al., 2020. Knowledge discovery with machine learning for hospital-acquired catheter-associated urinary tract infections. Comput. Inform. Nurs. 38 (1), 28–35. https://doi.org/10.1097/CIN.0000000000000562.

Russell, S.J., Stuart, J., Norvig, P., et al., 2022. Artificial Intelligence: A Modern Approach, fourth ed. Pearson, Hoboken, NJ.

Samoili, S., López Cobo, M., Gómez, E., et al., 2020. AI watch. Defining artificial intelligence: towards an operational definition and taxonomy of artificial intelligence. EUR 30117 EN. Publications Office of the European Union, Luxembourg, p. 2020. Available at: https://publications.jrc.ec.europa.eu/repository/bitstream/JRC118163/jrc118163_ai_watch._defining_artificial_intelligence_1.pdf.

World Health Organization, 2021. Ethics and governance of artificial intelligence for health. Available at: https://www.who.int/publications/i/item/9789240029200.

CHAPTER 16

Genomics and the Digital Revolution

Tracie Miles ■ J. Williams

LEARNING OUTCOMES

At the end of this chapter, the nurses will be able to :

- Have an overview of the rapid changes from genetics to genomics in recent decades.
- Understand the role of nursing in mainstreaming genomic testing when appropriate as opposed to the traditional model via clinical genetics.
- Have a critical awareness of the opportunities for digital technologies to support the advancement of genomics in clinical practice.
- Have a critical awareness of the organisational factors that support mainstreaming of genomics consultations.

Introduction

Generation Genome was born in the digital native age. The clinical community is learning to combine digital literacy with genomic literacy in healthcare to improve and enhance patient and family healthcare experience and options.

Genomics is transforming healthcare. For example, in cancer care, the use of targeted treatments has risen across the country (Bowel Cancer UK 2023). Over the next decade, targeted treatments for other common conditions, such as heart disease, dermatitis, and asthma, are expected to increase. Screening programmes to detect pathogenic genetic variants that can identify those at a higher risk of developing certain health issues before symptom onset and precision medicine for symptom management are also expected to become available (Calzone and Tonkin 2022). Simultaneously, the accelerating use of artificial intelligence (AI)-based technologies will transform genetic data into clinically useful information (Dias 2019).

There is an increasing awareness amongst the general population regarding how our genes, passed on through families, determine characteristics, such as hair colour and height, and influence our health. Traditionally, clinical care teams refer to specialist colleagues to provide genetic counselling and there is limited understanding of genomics amongst the general nurse population. However, realising the full range of benefits of genomics over the next 20 years will require all nurses to have a sufficient understanding of genomics and data science as part of mainstream clinical care.

Since the completion of mapping the *human genome* in 2003 (Lander et al. 2001; Gates et al. 2021), the global knowledge of how to harness the growing wealth of health information it brings is moving at pace. We are currently in a global 'generation genome' (Davies 2017), where discoveries to support health and wellbeing are being reported almost daily. As a result of this increased awareness, large sectors of the global community have become familiar with genomic terminology; for example, the concept of 'variants' during the Covid-19 pandemic, with the testing, tracing, and formulation of vaccines relying on digital and genomic knowledge combined to bring humanity out of the situation at pace.

Genomic information has the potential to support the implementation of targeted population-health screening (Ziff and Harris 2022), covering a wide range of disease or pre-disease states (Goldberg et al. 2011; National Institute of Health and Care Excellence (NICE) 2012), to maintain or improve population health and wellbeing.

Genomic data is increasingly used to enhance treatment planning, known as the companion or *test-to-treat principle.* Examples of this include precision medicine and targeted treatments in ovarian and breast cancer care (Hockings 2022).

In addition to cancer treatments, using digital solutions to create regional, national, and international databases of people with genomic risk-inheritance syndromes could dramatically improve global health. Inherited cardiac conditions, renal disease, familial hypercholesterolemia and monogenic diabetes are all examples where increased understanding of genomics can influence treatments and screening to enhance the health profile of individuals and populations.

As genomic testing evolves, providing more actionable data in both treatment and in continuing research (van Campen et al. 2019), the healthcare workforce is looking outside the traditional model of clinical genetics to provide genomic testing across all healthcare situations, to include health and wellbeing as well as ill health.

Mainstreaming Genomic Testing – Expanding the Role of the Nurse and Midwife

The need to offer genomic testing to patients across many disease states and to aid diagnosis and/or treatment requires clinical teams, including nurses and midwives, to initiate and facilitate such testing. This has been termed 'mainstreaming' (Hallowell et al. 2019) and incorporates pre-test genomic counselling and obtaining consent by a member of the clinical team caring for the patient (Georgiou et al. 2023).

The testing of a patient with a disease state is termed diagnostic testing, whereas the testing of a family member without the disease is termed pre-symptomatic testing. This point-of-care approach to genetic testing is not a completely novel concept to nursing and midwifery and has been used in some specific cases for some time (e.g. screening midwives counsel and obtain consent from expectant mothers for Down syndrome and sickle-cell anaemia). As testing molecular bio-markers becomes a routine part of the range of tests offered to patients, several oncology diagnostic workup pathways are becoming mainstream. The move away from clinical genetics-led testing to mainstreaming is fiscally advantageous and provides continuity of knowledge for both clinicians and patients (Georgiou et al. 2023). A seminal study on implementing routine genomic testing in patients with ovarian cancer (White et al. 2020) produced excellent outcomes in rapid, robust, cost-effective output in combination with high patient satisfaction. These principles have been transferred and scaled up to other tumour sites (e.g. breast, colorectal and endometrial) and across national and international services. A decade later, a systematic review addressing the feasibility of implementing mainstreaming in cancer care supports these outcomes (Badzek et al. 2013).

Genomic medicine and testing must be introduced in a way that is inclusive and equitable for both people and staff. Nurses need the knowledge and competence to provide appropriate information and care to individuals, families and communities, and to respond to potentially complex genomic issues (Badzek et al. 2013). Precision medicine has enormous potential to enhance public health but may have negative financial repercussions for people, like in securing life insurance policies. Access to this recent technology will need to be expanded equitably so that people do not experience variations based on geographical locations. Precision medicine will become increasingly significant to public health as the population continues to age, requiring nurses to interpret both avoidable and unavoidable disease risk factors for patients and their families.

While some aspects of genomics will remain within the remit of specialists, many others are being embedded in routine healthcare delivery. The nursing workforce plays a key role in efficiently, appropriately, and equitably utilising genomic testing, supporting people in understanding how their health may be affected based on genetic information. Research into the genetic basis of diseases and how best to support individuals and families through testing and decision-making is likely to become part of the working lives of an increasing number of nurses.

Within as little as five years, nurses will be routinely having discussions with patients regarding genomics and its impact upon health. This has the potential for nurses to address individualised health concerns and refer individuals to specialist screening programmes as required and indicated by specific guidelines. They will need to be supported by increased capacity and capability to investigate the use of precision medicine, including through audit, quality improvement and research. The Global Genomics Nursing Alliance (G2NA 2023) has influenced initial thinking in relation to integrating genomics into nursing practice. In UK, the seven regional NHS Genomic Medicine Services Alliances (GMSAs) (Hill 2020) bring together multi-professional clinical teams who have nurses embedded at strategic and operational levels to ensure that education and teaching include views of nurses and midwives.

Potentially, in the longer term, we can expect to see genomic data in electronic health records (EHRs) as standard, with whole-genome sequencing being offered more frequently to a wider range of individuals. As a result, people may be offered the option of learning about genomic risk factors of developing common conditions, such as heart disease, stroke and dementia. Nurses will need to understand the complex management of this data to ensure that any information shared is done so with the patient's permission. Clinicians should advocate for the appropriate inclusion of genomics data within EHR systems in procurement conversations with suppliers. Equally, suppliers need to focus on clinical engagement to ensure that systems have the necessary capabilities, and that the user interface is suited to the needs of the workforce. Nurses will also need to be trained in how to accurately collect and input data into an EHR system to ensure it meets the required standards for research and future innovation. Evidence suggests that this training is best delivered by fellow clinicians (Beyer 2022). To optimise patient safety, EHR systems that support decision-making must be subject to clinical safety approval, present data in an accessible way, and not override clinical judgement. Nurses with a confident command of data interpretation and analysis will also be able to provide transgenerational genetic counselling. They will consider environmental factors when planning treatment for people and aim to facilitate the delivery of this treatment in the most appropriate setting for the individual.

ESSENTIALS FOR SETTING UP A NURSE-LED MAINSTREAMING PATHWAY

- Genomic literacy of clinical team, including nurses with bespoke training/education programmes.
- A basic understanding of the ethical, legal and social issues of genomics in healthcare.
- Job planning of nurses to include discussions about genomic testing and consenting for these tests.
- Pathway mapping of mainstream service, to include timing, specimen collection, discussion and consent for testing, return of results, recording of results and referral to clinical genetics if appropriate.

Multidisciplinary collaboration is essential to these recommendations when mapping the mainstreaming pathway. This should involve a multidisciplinary clinical team plus clinical genetics advice and input and, most importantly, involve the patient's voice to review information support and accept a certain approach.

Preparing Nurses for Genomics

To this end, nurses will need a broad understanding of genomics, including in the context of precision medicine, family histories, and referral pathways. This learning should begin at pre-registration education, and genomics training should be mandatory for registered nurses as part of their practice to ensure there is no knowledge gap. Genomics is already part of specialist education pathways, such as oncology and cancer medicine, where shared decision-making with people using personalised medicine is already in use. However, it will become increasingly commonplace in a wider range of specialties.

As genomics rapidly evolves from a niche area to a necessity, education programmes need to be regularly updated to remain current. They are also more likely to have an impact when nurse experts are involved in their development. A roadmap for the future of nursing training in genomics will need to be adaptable to reflect the rapid and continual evolution of this technology in healthcare.

Because it emerged during the pandemic and because of the growing use of digital platforms to support learning, education for enhancing genomic knowledge for nurses at the novice as well as the expert level, is almost entirely online. An example of this is the Health Education England Genomic Education Programme, which provides a portfolio of learning opportunities for the multiprofessional workforce since its inception in 2020, with online courses being viewed 7,000,000 times. It provides leadership in this area, continuing to build digital and data literacy education programmes and incorporate these components into regulatory standards (Nursing & Midwifery Council 2018). Its e-learning courses, such as Genomics 101, which teaches health and care professionals with limited or no exposure to genomics in their clinical roles the fundamental principles of genomics and its applications in healthcare (Genomics Education Programme, 2023), have demonstrated positive results. As genomics knowledge grows, its dissemination via the worldwide web and social media alongside the conventional scientific/academic routes is increasing. It follows that the education requirements of today's nurse needs to move with this information tsunami to enable them to translate it into patient care. If nurses are involved with the development of learning packages, the uptake and understanding of content will be enhanced (Tonkin et al. 2020).

The GMSAs in England are at the forefront of genomics education work, sharing the concepts of its inception and process globally. Educating the multidisciplinary workforce is a key element of its work, with a growing digitally accessible portfolio of courses for learners at all levels on the Genomics Education Programme website. In addition to education, the NHS GMSA model provides a national model for nursing leadership and research, with multidisciplinary networks of excellence that are sharing their concepts and outputs globally. Furthermore, the active G2NA offers education and peer support across national boundaries.

LEARNING EXERCISE

Visit the Health Education England and Global Genomic Nursing Alliance websites to explore opportunities for expanding your knowledge of genomics:
  Home (g2na.org)
  Welcome to Genomics Education Programme – Genomics Education Programme (hee.nhs.uk)

The Intersection Between Advances in Genomic Science and Digital Technologies

Genomics and AI are identified as two of the digital advancements most likely to impact healthcare delivery in the next 20 years (Topol 2019). Together, they provide the opportunity for precision medicine, as genome sequencing data can be more widely interpreted and utilised for guiding healthcare for individuals.

AI can be described as technology in which computer systems perform tasks that would normally require human intelligence. Due to the sheer volume of data generated by whole-genome sequencing, genomics and the interpretation of this data are ideal areas of AI development.

There are already AI algorithms in development for variant calling, wherein the variants within an individual's genome are identified and further developed for AI classification. If AI is safely able to classify variants, there is the potential for whole-genome sequencing results to be fed back to patients in a shorter timeframe. There are limitations to the use of AI in variant calling and it will take a considerable amount of time for AI systems to become commonplace in clinical genomics.

Chapter 8 highlighted the need to identify secure clinical engagement stakeholders in the implementation of EHRs. This extends to genomics specialists to ensure data can be captured and repurposed for mainstream genomics practice. As organisations consider EHR integration the solution to effective and safe record-keeping, there is a further potential that digital governance can help in, with genomics being a 'family affair': the results of genomic tests may potentially hold information affecting family health and wellbeing. As a result, clinical genetics departments hold databases of inherited risk predisposition syndromes and rare disease. It is, therefore, essential that genomic results uploaded to the EHR are communicated to clinical geneticists where relevant. For example, a positive result may mean that family members of the patient tested by mainstreaming need to be offered cascade testing as they are at risk of having inherited the same genetic variant.

The genomic conversation with a patient (and family) is part of a continuum of conversation(s). It is not uncommon for patients and families to forget or be unsure of providing family history information during initial consults with their healthcare team. It may be during other care episodes that a patient remembers an important element of family history for record-keeping. Nurses across all care settings will need to understand where in the EHR family history records and genomic results can be located and act on this data, annotating if new information is provided by the patient. Furthermore, in their role as advocates, they will need to have sufficient knowledge to support people in understanding the implications of their genomic data on their decisions about lifestyle and treatment.

Digital technology in the form of apps will be a useful adjunct in enabling them fulfil this role. Apps can provide clinical decision-making support to enable identifying the effective triage of patients' eligibility for genomic testing and risk assessment, in line with guidelines relevant to the clinical community and published literature. An example of this is QGenome, developed by the Guy and St. Thomas' NHS Foundation Trust Regional Genetics Service and other NHS partners. QGenome enables point-of-care assessment to offer timely and efficient genomic testing in the patient pathway, thus facilitating quicker access to enhanced surveillance risk-reduction options, genetic counselling and testing for patients and their families. A further example of an online tool is CanRisk, which helps healthcare professionals calculate future risks of the development of breast and ovarian cancer, after reviewing family history, genetics and other risk factors.

Apps are also being developed to include up-to-date information support from both clinical and charitable sector providers. Examples include the MySunrise app from the NHS and The Eve Appeal mobile-ready information on genetic testing in ovarian cancer. Additionally, digital technology also provides the ability to send to patients digital family history questionnaires ahead of consultations to enhance the genomic conversation. It is important that nurses become acquainted and comfortable with these digital tools, used by clinical colleagues and the patient population alike, as they become embedded to their patient population care pathways.

The Chief Nursing Information Officer has a key role to play in ensuring that digital systems and tools support effective data capture, information retrieval, and transfer, including genomics data. They must act as a conduit between subject matter experts, system builders, and those supporting new ways of working. This is described in the case study below.

LEARNING EXERCISE

Consider how genomic data is integrated into EHRs in your organisation. Seek out colleagues to explore opportunities and collaborate.

LEARNING EXERCISE

Identify the lead nurse/midwife in your regional Genomic Medicine Service Alliance or local genetics service and contact them. Consider how you might share expertise and learning.

CASE STUDY: BREAST CANCER GENES AND ME

The genetic testing of a patient affected with breast cancer is usually the remit of the clinical genetics service. However, with the increase in therapeutic options and the requirement of test results during diagnostic workup, the mainstream approach to testing has the potential to provide more efficient personalised care. Consequently, the NHS England Southwest Genomic Medicine Service Alliance introduced a mainstreaming approach to *BRCA* gene testing on the diagnostic breast cancer pathway.

Taking a codesign approach, the solution was informed by patients, clinicians and technical experts and prior learning from an evaluation of the concept of digital consultations. A partnership grant was secured to fund the project, which attracted industry expertise. Assessment criteria included interoperability for effective information flows and workflows. Bringing together the expertise of the Regional Genomic Clinical Nurse Specialist and the Chief Nursing Information Officers in hospitals in the region was invaluable to secure the best solution that utilised digital technologies at the most appropriate points in the pathway. An additional benefit of this nursing leadership was that the clinical and patient engagement was secured.

Digital providers with a proven record of accomplishment with the NHS were invited to pitch a digital solution/platform to facilitate the virtual mainstreaming consultation, send the animation information to patients, complete relevant request forms and integrate results in the EHR. The result is a diagnostic pathway with flexible digital and non-digital workflows to suit individual patient needs; the digital animation can be used on its own or in combination with the counsel and consent consultation element attached to the EHR.

The digital **BReast CAncer Genes and Me** package was delivered in two parts: the digital patient information animation and the digital consultation, where the patient chooses one or both elements. The digital animation can be shared with the patient ahead of a digital consultation to counsel and obtain consent for the genomic test. Importantly, as genomics is very much a 'family affair', having a digital information resource means the patient can choose to share information easily with family members who are not in their immediate locality and invite family members to their online consultation if they so wish.

Evaluation shows positive feedback from patients and clinicians alike. These include:

- The ability to reach out to family members with the electronic information and consultation. This is always an important consideration but especially so in cases that have a potentially direct impact on family members, depending on the patient's result.
- The ability to have a digitally enabled remote consultation to cut down on mental, physical and financial costs of travelling when the patient is already overloaded with appointments during the intense diagnostic cancer pathway and early treatment phase.
- The continued maintenance of caregiver communication, celebrated repeatedly by patients.

An example video of patient feedback (Video16.1) and the animation (Video 16.2) are hosted on Evolve: http://evolve.elsevier.com/Phillips/digital/

Conclusion

This chapter has highlighted how genomics, coupled with rapid advancements in the use of digital technologies, can enable improved individual and population health outcomes. It has indicated the implications for practice and the education of nurses, introducing resources to support further learning. Key factors that affect the successful adoption of new knowledge and technologies have been discussed and supported with a case study and learning exercises to enable the reader to consider application to practice.

Key Points

1. Genomics is advancing rapidly and has the potential to significantly improve outcomes and improve population health through precision medicine.
2. Providing nurses with education in genomics relevant to their practice is essential to realise the benefits of genomic science.
3. Seeking support from non-healthcare providers as partner stakeholders to advance the technologies efficiently together (providing complimentary skillsets) is crucial.
4. Patients and the public have a key role to play in the design and development of mainstreamed genomic services.

References

Badzek, L., Henaghan, M., Turner, T., et al., 2013. Ethical, legal, and social issues in the translation of genomics into health care. J. Nurs. Scholarsh. 45 (1), 15–24.

Beyer, A., 2022. Trust in organization/IT leadership 2022. Available at: https://klasresearch.com/archcollaborative/report/trust-in-organization-it-leadership-2022/425.

Bowel Cancer UK, 2023. Mo Haque, London Available at: https://www.bowelcanceruk.org.uk/how-we-can-help/real-life-stories/younger-people-with-bowel-cancer/mo-haque,-35-from-london/.

Calzone, K.A., Tonkin, E., 2022. Genomic education and training resources for nursing. In: Kumar, D. (Ed.), Genomic Medicine Skills and Competencies. Elsevier, London.

Davies, S.C., 2017. Annual Report of the Chief Medical Officer 2016: Generation Genome. Department of Health and Social Care, London.

Dias, R., Torkamani, A., 2019. Artificial intelligence in clinical and genomic diagnostics. Genome Med. 11 (1), 70.

Gates, A.J., Gysi, D.M., Kellis, M., et al., 2021. A wealth of discovery built on the Human Genome Project – by the numbers. Nature 590 (7845), 212–215.

Genomics Education Programme, 2023. Genomics 101. Available at: https://www.genomicseducation.hee.nhs.uk/product-tag/genomics-101/.

Georgiou, D., Monje-Garcia, L., Miles, T., et al., 2023. A focused clinical review of Lynch syndrome. Cancer Manag. Res. 15, 67–85.

Goldberg, A.C., Hopkins, P.N., Toth, P.P., et al., 2011. Familial hypercholesterolemia: screening, diagnosis and management of pediatric and adult patients: clinical guidance from the National Lipid Association Expert Panel on Familial Hypercholesterolemia. J. Clin. Lipidol. 5 (3 Suppl. l), 133–140.

Hallowell, N., Wright, S., Stirling, D., et al., 2019. Moving into the mainstream: healthcare professionals' views of implementing treatment focussed genetic testing in breast cancer care. Fam. Cancer 18 (3), 293–301.

Hill, S., 2020. NHS Genomic Medicine Service Alliances to Help Embed Genomics into Patient Care Pathways. Available at: https://www.england.nhs.uk/blog/nhs-genomic-medicine-service-alliances-to-help-embed-genomics-into-patient-care-pathways/.

Hockings, H., 2022. PARP Inhibitors. Available at: https://www.genomicseducation.hee.nhs.uk/genotes/knowledge-hub/parp-inhibitors/.

Lander, E.S., Linton, L.M., Birren, B., et al., 2001. Initial sequencing and analysis of the human genome. Nature 409 (6822), 860–921.

National Institute of Health and Care Excellence (NICE), 2012. Familial Hypercholesterolaemia Genetic Screening Clinics. Available at: https://www.nice.org.uk/sharedlearning/familial-hypercholesterolaemia-genetic-screening-clinics.

NHS England, 2022. Accelerating Genomic Medicine in the NHS. Available at: https://www.england.nhs.uk/long-read/accelerating-genomic-medicine-in-the-nhs/.

NursingMidwifery Council (NMC), 2018. Future Nurse: Standards of Proficiency for Registered Nurses. Available at: https://www.nmc.org.uk/globalassets/sitedocuments/education-standards/future-nurse-proficiencies.pdf.

Tonkin, E., Calzone, K.A., Badzek, L., et al., 2020. A roadmap for global acceleration of genomics integration across nursing. J. Nurs. Scholarsh. 52 (3), 329–338.

Topol, E.J., 2019. Preparing the Healthcare Workforce to Deliver the Digital Future: An Independent Report on Behalf of the Secretary of State for Health and Social Care. Health Education England, London. February 2019.

van Campen, J.C., Sollars, E.S.A., Thomas, R.C., et al., 2019. Next generation sequencing in newborn screening in the United Kingdom National Health Service. Int. J. Neonatal Screen 5 (4), 40.

White, S., Jacobs, C., Phillips, J., 2020. Mainstreaming genetics and genomics: a systematic review of the barriers and facilitators for nurses and physicians in secondary and tertiary care. Genet. Med. 22 (7), 1149–1155.

Ziff, M., Harris, J., 2022. A collaborative genetic carrier screening model for the British Ashkenazi Jewish community. J. Community Genet. 13 (1), 133–135.

CHAPTER 17

Remote Care and Virtual Wards: Transforming Nursing Practice

Emily Wells

LEARNING OUTCOMES

At the end of this chapter, the nurses will be able to:

- Understand the concept of remote care and virtual wards and their relevance to nursing practice.
- Examine the key elements involved in transforming traditional face-to-face health and care models into virtual care models.
- Differentiate between the various digital technologies and data tools that underpin remote care and virtual wards.
- Identify the core skills and competencies required by nurses to lead and participate in virtual care transformation.
- Consider the benefits and challenges associated with implementing remote care and virtual wards in nursing practice.

Introduction

The rapid advancements in digital technology and data are continuing to transform healthcare globally. One key aspect of this transformation is the shift towards remote care and virtual wards, which is replacing traditional hospital-based care models with care and treatment at home. Examples include the use of video consultations and remote physiological monitoring, enabling hospital teams to replace face-to-face outpatient and in-patient care. This chapter discusses the importance of remote care and virtual wards in the current health and care climate as well as the role of nurses in leading this form of digital innovation. It also considers the challenges and practical implications for nursing practice, including core knowledge and skills. Whilst there is some evidence that providing care in a virtual setting is equal to standard care, with some outcomes for specific conditions such as heart failure being greatly improved (Chauhan and McAlister 2022) there are still some uncertainties about their long-term impact on quality, safety, performance, outcomes and experience of people and the people who care for them. This chapter presents a pragmatic approach for the development of virtual care and identifies key areas for consideration when virtual care models are being developed and delivered.

Overview

Remote care and virtual wards represent a paradigm shift in healthcare delivery, where acute care is provided to patients in their homes or other non-hospital settings, supported through digital technology and data management tools. In the NHS in England, the key elements of virtual ward provision have been defined as:

- Providing acute care and treatment at home
- Developing treatment plan for an acute problem (not long-term condition management)
- Naming responsible clinician
- Daily review of progress by multidisciplinary team (as guided by treatment plan)
- Using technology as an adjunct to care; that is, video consultations and/or remote physiological monitoring through the use of wearable technology
- Avoiding in-patient admission completely or shortening a necessary in-patient hospital stay (NHS England 2022)

Other types of remote care use either telephone or video calls to contact patients, replacing face-to-face appointments in primary care and outpatient departments. Additionally, intermittent physiological monitoring and the use of patient-reported outcomes entered into apps or websites are being used for long-term condition management; these can also be used to monitor patients for early signs of disease progression or acute deterioration. However, the lack of clear and consistent definitions for remote care and virtual ward models has been confusing for staff, patients and families as services have rapidly evolved. Hospital-at-Home models for older patients and those with long-term conditions, for example, have been in place for many years. These models contain many of the elements of a virtual ward by delivering hospital level care at a person's home and avoiding in-patient admission.

Despite challenges with definitions and different service models, virtual wards have significant advantages over traditional care models. For example, patients living in rural or remote areas can access healthcare services more easily, and patients receiving remote care have reduced hospitalisations and re-admissions (Buyting et al. 2022; Dolan et al. 2021; Gonclaves-Bradley et al. 2017). Because patients are receiving care in a more familiar and comfortable environment, they can maintain their autonomy and involvement in their care. In addition, they have a reduced risk of the iatrogenic consequences of hospitalisation, such as hospital-acquired infection, falls and delirium. All these factors mean that outcomes for patients may improve.

For nurses working in remote care or virtual wards, there is the opportunity to provide more personalised and patient-centred care and support patient empowerment. This requires nurses to develop new clinical skills that combine the unique caring skills of the profession with the use of technology to monitor patients' health and wellbeing. The development and implementation of innovative care models can also provide opportunities to collaborate with other healthcare professionals in an interdisciplinary team and have a more flexible approach to working.

TRANSFORMATIONAL BUILDING BLOCKS FOR VIRTUAL CARE MODELS

There are several elements to consider when implementing virtual care models in an established clinical service (Table 17.1). These include a range of strategic, clinical, operational, financial, data, as well as digital and engagement principles and processes to agree, codesign and operationalise to maximise the opportunities for successful implementation.

Shifting acute care from hospital to home supported by technology requires visible senior clinical leadership and the ability for leaders and teams to constantly evolve services based on their quality, safety, performance and outcomes data, together with the emerging evidence.

TABLE 17.1 ■ Elements to Consider for Implementing Virtual Care Models

Area	Elements
Strategic	Executive sponsorship Features within strategic direction of the organisation Commitment to embedding codesign at all levels
Clinical	Clinical governance arrangements including identified clinical lead for the service Policies and procedures for monitoring quality, safety, experience and outcomes Clinical pathways, including admission and discharge criteria, referral routes and escalation processes Build pathways into workflows Identify multidisciplinary workforce to manage caseload Training and development plan and approach
Operational	Operating processes and procedures, including arrangements for support from existing services (e.g. diagnostics, community team) Identifying operational lead Providing project management support
Financial	Agreed-upon recurrent funding model for workforce and technology Benefits management and return on investment plan
Data and digital	Agreed data collection method and approach, including reporting Outcomes measurement plan Technology selection that ensures patient, carer and staff needs are optimally met Digital clinical safety management
Engagement	Strategic communication plan and campaign across all interfacing organizations Continuous engagement and codesign with patients, carers and families

Adapted from Thomas et al. (2021).

DIGITAL TECHNOLOGIES AND DATA MANAGEMENT IN REMOTE CARE AND VIRTUAL WARDS

Several digital technologies and data management tools underpin remote care and virtual wards, including telehealth, remote monitoring devices, mobile health applications, electronic health records (EHRs) and the use of data analytics tools. Telehealth platforms facilitate real-time communication between patients and healthcare providers, allowing for virtual consultations, assessments and monitoring. Being able to 'see' the patient (and often their home environment) is a critical element that supports decision-making when providing virtual care (Nagel et al. 2016).

Remote monitoring devices enable patients to monitor their vital signs, symptoms and other health indicators at home, with the data transmitted to healthcare providers for review and analysis. These devices commonly monitor heart rate, respiratory rate, temperature, blood pressure and oxygen saturation. Some data platforms enable 'alerts' to be set that trigger when agreed parameters have been breached. Activity levels can also be monitored via a step count. Additionally, weighing scales with Bluetooth connectivity can also support the care of patients with heart failure, for example. Remote monitoring using point-of-care testing and novel diagnostics has almost infinite potential with the ability to carry out urinalysis, capillary blood glucose and C-reactive protein and capillary blood ketone levels. Such devices can provide continuous or intermittent data that is automatically transmitted or entered into a specific app by the patient/carer. Patients are also able to report their symptoms, current functional status and concerns if that functionality is part of the monitoring device. In addition, mobile health applications provide patients with access to health information, resources and tools to manage their health and wellbeing. They can also be used in acute illness to monitor for signs of deterioration, such as low oxygen saturation during coronavirus infection (Houlding et al. 2021) as well as for monitoring chronic illness (Alvarez et al. 2021).

EHRs facilitate the storage, retrieval and sharing of patient information, enabling healthcare providers to make more informed decisions and coordinate care more effectively. Shared care records/health information exchanges link EHRs and other patient data systems, such as pathology and radiology, to enable wider data sharing between primary, secondary, tertiary and social care. Data analytics tools allow healthcare providers to collect and analyse patient data, identify trends and make data-informed decisions to improve patient outcomes. Data collection must be standardised to ensure consistency in measurement between staff, over time and across services. Analytics can support patient-level decision-making as well as whole-service evaluation.

LEARNING EXERCISE

a) List the digital technologies in use and identify their functionalities.
b) What functionalities are available? Are they used maximally by all staff?
c) How does the technology interface with any existing systems and what are the operational challenges?
d) Do all staff providing remote care have access to the technology? Are any workarounds in place?

CORE SKILLS AND COMPETENCIES FOR NURSES IN REMOTE CARE AND VIRTUAL WARDS

To lead and participate in digital transformation to remote care provision, nurses need a set of skills and competencies, including proficiency in using digital technologies and data management tools, to deliver remote care, communicate with patients and collaborate with other healthcare professionals. This also includes understanding the limitations of the digital systems being used; for example, a lack of interoperability between different systems can create fragmented or missing patient information (Nagel et al. 2016). In addition, the ability to make evidence-based decisions is crucial in remote care and virtual wards, as nurses must be able to analyse patient data, identify trends and adapt care plans accordingly. Being able to 'see' the patients and visually observe them for prolonged periods is not possible. Nurses must be cognisant of any risks associated with the limitations of virtual care and escalate appropriately. Nurses and midwives must understand the quality, safety, outcomes and performance data of their services. Their knowledge of how services are delivered, together with detailed data analysis, will enable them to have a comprehensive understanding of the benefits, risks and challenges. The use of quality improvement methods and data to measure the impact of any service change will add to the local evidence base and increase confidence in new services and demonstrate the value.

It is vital to ensure that the care provided remotely is inclusive. Nurses are well placed to identify those patients who can optimally benefit from remote care but also those who are at risk of poorer access (Fotis 2022). Patients and carers with poor digital skills or limited internet access are likely to be the most disadvantaged in terms of equitable access to this type of care (Sieck et al. 2021). Nurses are in a unique position to understand access challenges locally and work with partner organisations to increase inclusivity. Nurses must prioritise patient needs, preferences and values, fostering patient autonomy and involvement in their care. Virtual care provides another opportunity to embed shared decision-making into care planning, ensuring that patient goals and wishes are a central focus (NHS England 2019).

Nurses are already skilled in working effectively with other healthcare professionals, both within their own discipline and across disciplines. The delivery of remote care and virtual wards requires even further integration between primary care staff, hospital-based teams and community services. Nurses can play a pivotal role in building trust and collegiate relationships, as teams not used to working in this way work together to develop virtual care pathways. The rapidly evolving nature of digital technology and healthcare requires nurses to be adaptable and innovative in their approach to remote care and virtual wards, embracing new technologies, care models and best practices as they emerge. Nurses must play an active role in the development of virtual care models to ensure, as they evolve, that the users' and patients' needs and requirements are highlighted and adequately addressed.

In the UK, a core skills and capabilities framework has been developed for virtual ward staff to support the provision of high-quality personalised care using technology. The framework can also support training programmes, personal development planning, career progression and workforce models (Skills for Health 2022).

BENEFITS AND CHALLENGES OF REMOTE CARE AND VIRTUAL WARDS

While remote care and virtual wards have the potential to offer numerous benefits for patients, families and nursing practice, they also present certain challenges. Virtual care should not be adopted in an uncritical way. Remote care is not a panacea for all current challenges with health and care delivery. Optimising service delivery requires a flexible yet sustained approach to unblocking challenges, using robust data and quality improvement methods to monitor the impact of changes.

The provision of remote care and virtual wards needs a skilled workforce and there are international challenges in both recruiting and retaining nurses. Whilst providing remote care might be an attractive option for some nurses, overall, the relatively small pool of staff is likely to create depletion in other areas. Some posts may be especially hard to recruit for and require a long-term strategy to build future workforce requirements. Once recruited, staff require training and supervision to develop the requisite knowledge and skills for remote care delivery. This requires a training and competency assessment infrastructure which will take time to develop. The workforce is also a critical part of the programme and project team to ensure that services are codesigned with those delivering them as they are developed. In addition, there may be some resistance to reframing how acute care is delivered.

Hospital-based acute care has been well established for hundreds of years and healthcare professionals are trained based on care delivery in these traditional models. Remote care and virtual wards fundamentally change care models for some acute illnesses and the traditional ward-based connection with patients and staff no longer exists. There are genuine concerns about quality, safety, outcomes and the clinical roles that have accountability and responsibility as services rapidly expand; these need to be considered when transforming a service.

There are also challenges regarding peoples' access to digital technologies and high-speed internet, which is not universal. While some technologies do not require people to have their own internet access, all individuals receiving care will require some degree of input to enable them to be supported remotely. Remote services will need to develop infrastructures that can provide people and families with technical support on admission and during their treatment, ideally over a 24-hour period 7 days a week. Linked to issues of access to technology is an understanding of potential issues related to digital exclusion. Comprehensive equality impact assessments are the first step in understanding when, how and why some of the population may be prevented or limited in accessing remote care. Citizens with other vulnerabilities (e.g. sensory impairments) will require an additional support infrastructure to enable access to remote care. Provision of technologies in a range of languages and media, tailored to the needs of the local communities is essential. There needs to be an unwavering commitment to ensuring equitable access and close monitoring of patient demographics to understand where further targeted support is needed.

Some groups in local communities already experience health inequalities due to poor access and uptake of or traditional face-to-face services. Understanding the challenges for these groups and the staff providing services can give further insight into the requirements for virtual care.

Data security and privacy is also a key issue when establishing remote care and virtual wards. A thorough understanding of the relevant data protection legislation is required to ensure that the processing and storage of patient data is lawful. Robust policies, procedures and training of staff are required to ensure that the legislation is understood and adhered to. Patients and families should have easily accessible information about how their data is stored and used. Patients expect healthcare staff to have access to all their health information when they are receiving direct care. How patient data may be used for service planning and research is generally less well understood by the public and opportunities to 'opt-out' of having patient data used in this way must be in place. Transparency is critical in creating trust between patients and services, so there is a complete understanding of how confidentiality is maintained and how patients can consent to supporting remote care research, if they so wish.

There has been a rapid expansion of remote monitoring products and the market has been flooded in recent years. Remote monitoring technology is a critical adjunct to care in the same way that hospital-based physiological monitoring is. Most remote monitoring technology offers the same physiological monitoring capabilities; however, it is important that product selection is based on staff, patients' and carers' needs and preferences. Crucial for staff is the integration of any new technology into existing information technology systems, ensuring that the full multidisciplinary team (whether hospital- or community-based) has access and can contribute to the full patient record. Patients and carers need products that have been codesigned and can be tailored to the condition, circumstances and preferences. They must be easy to use for those with additional needs and enable input from carers if required. Scoping a 'minimum viable product' from staff and patients' perspective is a critical first step in product selection. Additionally, manufacturers should offer flexible solutions that can be tailored to the needs of the services, committing to working with organisations and services to develop products that meet all the requirements from a digital and data-capture perspective.

As services rapidly develop, the established financial models for payment may not fit the new service design. With acute care moving from hospital to the community or the patient's own home, financial flows will need to replicate this shift in place of care to enable appropriate funding of the services. Delays in securing funding, especially in the current cost-restricted climate in many countries, can delay service transformation. Linked to financial models is clear evidence of cost-effectiveness and a comprehensive health economic evaluation, as services develop and expand. The development of datasets with agreed definitions is critical for consistent measurement and evaluation of services. This can enable a thorough understanding of the safety, quality and cost-effectiveness of services in comparison to traditional care models as well as understanding patient outcomes when managed remotely. Data and measurement should be a key workstream as services develop pooling the knowledge, skills and expertise of clinicians, patients, data analysts and information teams.

CASE STUDY: NORFOLK AND NORWICH VIRTUAL WARD

BACKGROUND

The Norfolk and Norwich Virtual Ward leverages digital technology to provide remote care for patients at home. By integrating telehealth, remote monitoring and data analytics, the virtual ward was established to provide safe and effective monitoring and a follow-up service for all patients, while facilitating early discharge, admission avoidance and physical bed-occupancy reduction, where possible and clinically safe. Expected benefits included improved patient experience and outcomes, reduced length of stay in an acute bed and more efficient delivery of healthcare.

The Norfolk and Norwich Virtual Ward was designed to provide a seamless transition between hospital and home-based care for patients, employing a multidisciplinary team of nurses, doctors, pharmacists and other healthcare professionals. The team works together to support patient needs, with regular virtual consultations and remote monitoring of vital signs and other relevant health data.

Key components of the Norfolk and Norwich Virtual Ward included:

- 24/7 model of care: Offering round-the-clock remote and continuous monitoring of patients, the ward operated 24 hours a day, 7 days a week, mirroring a physical in-patient ward.
- Patient selection: The multidisciplinary team identified patients with complex care needs who were at risk of frequent hospital admissions, based on factors such as previous hospitalization history, multiple comorbidities and socioeconomic status.
- Pathway design: For each pathway, the team developed a comprehensive, patient-centred plan that addressed specific needs, preferences and values. This plan was regularly reviewed and updated, as needed.
- Remote monitoring: Patients were provided with digital devices and wearables, such as blood pressure monitors, glucose meters and pulse oximeters, to track their vital signs and other health data remotely. This information was transmitted securely to the virtual ward team for review and analysis.
- Virtual consultations: The virtual ward team conducted daily (and more frequently, if necessary) video consultations with patients to assess their health, provide education and support and address any concerns or issues that arose. These consultations were scheduled based on each patient's needs and preferences, with additional consultations available as required.
- Interdisciplinary collaboration: The virtual ward team held daily virtual ward rounds to discuss patient cases, review health data and coordinate care. This collaboration helped ensure that all team members were informed about each patient's needs and progress and that any issues or complications were promptly addressed.

OUTCOMES AND LESSONS LEARNED

The Norfolk and Norwich Virtual Ward has proven successful in improving patient outcomes and enhancing patient satisfaction. Key outcomes and lessons learned from this initiative include:

- Improved patient outcomes: The virtual ward's focus on early intervention, prevention and patient education led to improved patient outcomes, such as better management of chronic conditions and fewer complications.
- Enhanced patient satisfaction: Patients reported high levels of satisfaction with the virtual ward, citing the convenience and accessibility of remote consultations, personalized care and the supportive relationship they developed with their healthcare team.
- Interdisciplinary collaboration: The close collaboration between the virtual ward team members, including nurses, midwives and other healthcare professionals,

---

CASE STUDY: NORFOLK AND NORWICH VIRTUAL WARD—cont'd

---

facilitated better care coordination and more comprehensive, holistic care for patients.
- The importance of digital literacy and continuous professional development: The success of the Norfolk and Norwich Virtual Ward underscored the need for healthcare professionals, including nurses and midwives, to develop digital literacy and invest in continuous professional development to effectively utilize digital technologies and data management tools in remote care and virtual ward settings.

By analysing the experiences and outcomes of the Norfolk and Norwich Virtual Ward, this case study provides valuable insights and recommendations for implementing remote care and virtual ward initiatives in nursing and midwifery practice, both in the UK and internationally.

Conclusion

Remote care and virtual wards are transforming the landscape of nursing practice, offering opportunities to improve healthcare access and enhance patient experience and outcomes. By developing the core skills and competencies required to lead and participate in digital transformation, and by learning from the experiences of other countries and healthcare systems, nurses have a crucial role to play in shaping the future of healthcare and driving the adoption of remote care and virtual wards. The lessons learned from the Norfolk and Norwich Virtual Ward case study and the broader literature on remote care and virtual wards provide valuable insights and recommendations for translating learning into practice and ensuring the successful implementation of remote care and virtual ward initiatives globally. As digital technologies and data management tools continue to advance, it is crucial for nurses to lead developments by staying informed, adapting care delivery and preparing for the future, ensuring that they remain at the forefront and play a key leadership role in this exciting and rapidly evolving field.

Key Points

1. Defining the scope of services and eligible patient cohorts is critical.
2. The evidence base for virtual wards and remote care is relatively immature. Virtual care models should not be adopted without caution and on-going evaluation, which involves ensuring that datasets are developed and regular measurement and reporting is in place.
3. Strategic communications are required across all settings to ensure that hospital and community-based teams understand these new services, identify eligible patients and understand how to refer these patients to virtual wards.
4. Codesign services with staff and patients ensuring close involvement from patients who have additional needs and may have limited access to digital systems or limited confidence in them.

References

Alvarez, P., Sianis, A., Brown, J., et al., 2021. Chronic disease management in heart failure: focus on telemedicine and remote monitoring. Rev. Cardiovasc. Med. 22 (2), 403–413.

Buyting, R., Melville, S., Chatur, H., White, C.W., Légaré, J.-F., Lutchmedial, S., Brunt, K.R., 2022. Virtual care with digital technologies for rural Canadians living with cardiovascular disease. CJC Open 4 (2), 133–147.

Chauhan, U., McAlister, F.A., 2022. Comparison of mortality and hospital readmissions among patients receiving virtual ward transitional care vs usual postdischarge care: a systematic review and meta-analysis. JAMA Netw. Open 5 (6), e2219113.

Dolan, H., Eggett, C., Holliday, L., Delves, S., Parkes, D., Sutherland, K., 2021. Virtual care in end of life and palliative care: a rapid evidence check. J. Telemed. Telecare 27 (10), 631–637.

Fotis, T., 2022. Digital nursing and health care innovation. J. Perianesthesia Nurs. 37 (1), 3–4. https://doi.org/10.1016/j.jopan.2021.11.006.

Goncalves-Bradley, D.C., Iliffe, S., Doll, H.A., et al., 2017. Early discharge hospital at home. Cochrane Database Syst. Rev. 2017 (6), CD000356.

Houlding, E., Mate, K.K.V., Engler, K., et al., 2021. Barriers to use of remote monitoring technologies used to support patients with COVID-19: rapid review. JMIR. Mhealth Uhealth 9 (4), e24743.

Nagel, D.A., Stacey, D., Momtahan, K., Gifford, W., Doucet, S., Etowa, J.B., 2016. Getting a picture: a grounded theory of nurses knowing the person in a virtual environment. J. Holist. Nurs. 35 (1), 67–85. https://doi.org/10.1177/08980 10116 645422.

NHS England, 2019. Shared Decision Making: Summary Guide. Available at: https://www.england.nhs.uk/wp-content/uploads/2019/01/shared-decision-making-summary-guide-v1.pdf.

NHS England, 2022. Supporting Information: Virtual Ward Including Hospital at Home. Available at: https://www.england.nhs.uk/wp-content/uploads/2021/12/B1478-supporting-guidance-virtual-ward-including-hospital-at-home-march-2022-update.pdf.

Skills for Health, 2022. Virtual Ward and Urgent Community Response Capabilities Framework. Available at: https://www.skillsforhealth.org.uk/wp-content/uploads/2022/09/VW-and-UCR-Capabilities-Framework-FINAL-290922-proofed-version-with-sigs.pdf.

Sieck, C.J., Sheon, A., Ancker, J.S., et al., 2021. Digital inclusion as a social determinant of health. NPJ. Digit. Med. 4, 52.

Thomas, E.E., Taylor, M.L., Banbury, A., et al., 2021. Factors influencing the effectiveness of remote patient monitoring interventions: a realist review. BMJ Open 11 (8), e051844.

Conclusion

We are facing a global workforce crisis, where attrition from the profession is attributed to poor workplace conditions, lack of time to engage in meaningful care interactions and an inability to ensure safe and effective service provision. We cannot ignore the enduring impact on the morale of the workforce and significant transformation to models of care is required.

Throughout this text, we, and our authors, have argued that we are embarking on a new age for nursing assisted and enabled by technology and data. Many of us are embracing this prospect, but others are sceptical and concerned about what this will mean for the future of how we deliver care, particularly the risks of digital exclusion and widening health inequalities. This book has described how the medium of technology and the power of data has the potential for nursing to utilise the science to enhance the art of practice, particularly our ability to personalise care to the individual, family, community and inform how we design services to promote the wellbeing of populations.

The digital transformation agenda in healthcare is moving at a rapid pace. The possibilities of emergent technologies for the enhancement of the quality and safety of care are both inspiring and overwhelming in equal measures. There is a danger that the experts in the technologies, digital system providers and other healthcare professionals will dictate the pace and potential of transformation and, as a result, the solutions will not be fit for purpose, nor will they serve the people and practitioners who will use them. As a profession, we simply cannot allow this to happen. The opportunity for digital to enable us to reconnect with the joy of practice will pass us by and we will lose the trust of our patients who are increasingly calling on us to be their partners and navigators of care. We must step into places of influence and use our unique nursing expertise to give us the authority to define and shape the agenda, rather than it being imposed upon us.

We acknowledge that in order to respond to this impetus for change, the digital literacy of our workforce will require significant development. This begins in the way we educate our pre-registration students and follows through to our established workforce where there is a wide breadth of confidence and trust in the digitally enabled care agenda. In the short term, there is a need for digital nursing leaders who are expert in both the technological opportunities and the ability to translate these into practice. These champions of digitally enabled care will provide the bridge and be a supportive guide to enable those less confident or sceptical to embrace new ways of working. In the longer term, we envisage a time when every nurse understands the potential of technology and data and every nurse considers digital as integral to their practice.

Looking to the future, we have a huge challenge but one we cannot ignore. Our hope is that this book has offered you valuable insights from digital health leaders and demonstrated the value of our professional voice in this space. We all have the potential to learn from them and consider how we can be equally transformational within our own spheres of influence.

We started our book with a definition of person-centred practice and the proposition that technology and data have the potential to enable this way of working across systems, services and within every care interaction. The outcome of this would be a healthful culture, described as one in which decision-making is shared, relationships are collaborative, leadership is transformational, and innovative practices are supported. Development of a healthful culture has the potential to create conditions that enable human flourishing for those who give and for those who receive care (McCormack et al. 2021). As nurses, it is these conditions that we always have, and always will, aspire to reach, and that is achievable by harnessing digital technology and data science.

References

McCormack, B., McCance, T., Brown, D., Bulley, C., McMillan, A., & Martin, S., 2021. Fundamentals of Person-centred Healthcare Practice. Wiley-Blackwell Publishing Ltd.

Note: Page numbers followed by *b* indicate boxes; *f*, figures; and *t*, tables.